The Complete

MEDITERRANEAN

Kids Diet Cookbook

Learn To Prepare Delicious, Budget Friendly, and Wholesome Meals Easily and Quickly with Step-by-Step Instruction

Etta William

FOR MORE INTERSTING BOOKS FROM THE AUTHOR KINDLY SCAN THE BARCODE BELOW

OR CLICK ON **HERE**

About Author

Etta William is a multi-talented British American author, nutritionist, and writer, known for her expertise in the fields of health, nutrition, diet, and cookbooks. Etta's journey in the world of nutrition and culinary arts began with her academic pursuits at the prestigious Massachusetts Institute of Technology (MIT), where she honed her knowledge and skills in various aspects of nutrition and healthy living.

As a seasoned nutritionist, Etta has dedicated her career to helping individuals make informed choices about their diets and overall well-being. Her passion for promoting healthy eating and lifestyles shines through in her work, where she combines scientific knowledge with a practical approach to guide readers and enthusiasts on their paths to better health.

Etta's commitment to her craft extends beyond her profession as a nutritionist. She has established herself as a prolific writer, with a particular focus on health, nutrition, and cookbooks. Her writing is not only informative but also highly accessible, making complex dietary concepts and recipes easily understandable to a broad audience.

Through her books, Etta shares her insights and recipes, aiming to inspire and empower readers to embrace a healthier way of life. Her cookbooks are a testament to her culinary prowess and her dedication to creating dishes that are both delicious and nutritious, providing readers with a wealth of options to nourish their bodies.

With a unique blend of scientific knowledge and a passion for good food, Etta William continues to make a significant impact in the world of health and nutrition. Her work serves as a valuable resource for those seeking to improve their dietary choices and embark on a journey towards better health and well-being. Etta's contributions as an author and nutritionist have undoubtedly enriched the lives of many, offering guidance and inspiration on the path to a healthier lifestyle.

Table of Content

Introduction

The Mediterranean Diet is well-known around the world for emphasizing healthful, nutrient-dense foods that are modeled after the customary eating habits of nations that border the Mediterranean Sea. This diet emphasizes heart-healthy fats, lean proteins, whole grains, fresh, unprocessed products, and a wide range of fruits and vegetables. It is more than just a list of meals to follow. Fundamentally, it advocates for a harmony between general health, flavor, and nutrition.

A. Overview of the Mediterranean Diet

A diet that emphasizes plant-based foods such as fruits, vegetables, nuts, legumes, whole grains, olive oil, and dairy in moderation, the Mediterranean Diet is known for its plant-based composition. It advocates for a high consumption of fiber and antioxidants from plant sources and is low in processed foods and red meat.

Consuming olive oil is essential to this diet, especially extra-virgin olive oil, which has a high concentration of antioxidants and monounsaturated fats that support the diet's cardio-protective properties. Another component of this diet is the moderate intake of wine, preferably red wine, which provides antioxidants like resveratrol.

B. Benefits of the Mediterranean Diet for Kids

Adopting the Mediterranean Diet has several health benefits for kids. Because of its high nutrient content, it provides vital vitamins, minerals, and antioxidants for healthy growth and development. The focus on whole meals improves metabolic health, lowers the risk of pediatric obesity, and helps people control their weight better.

Children's brain growth and cognitive performance are supported by the diet's emphasis on good fats, such as those in fish and olive oil. Including a variety of fruits and vegetables also promotes a higher nutrient intake, strengthening the immune system and enhancing general health.

C. How to Implement the Mediterranean Diet for Children

The Mediterranean diet must be introduced to kids gradually and inclusively. Promote a range of vibrant fruits and vegetables by arranging them in an eye-catching manner and involving yourself in meal planning and preparation. To promote healthier eating habits, swap out unhealthy snacks for almonds, seeds, or fresh fruit.

Reduce the intake of refined grains and increase the use of healthy grains such brown rice, quinoa, and whole wheat pasta. Give lean proteins (fish, poultry, lentils, nuts) priority and limit processed meats. Furthermore, stress the need of using olive oil as your main source of fat and for cooking.

D. Essential Ingredients and Cooking Techniques

A variety of vegetables, such as tomatoes, eggplants, spinach, and bell peppers, as well as olive oil—which is used as a main cooking fat and flavor enhancer—are essential components of the Mediterranean diet. Beans, lentils, and chickpeas are examples of legumes that offer a significant supply of fiber and protein. Whole grains give meals diversity and nutrition, such as barley, farro, and bulgur.

To preserve nutrients and enhance flavors, cooking procedures commonly involve grilling, roasting, or sautéing food in olive oil. Mediterranean cuisine has a distinct flavor profile that is enhanced by the use of fresh herbs such as parsley, basil, oregano, and thyme. Involve kids in kitchen activities to help them develop a respect for nutritious ingredients and cooking techniques.

This all-inclusive approach to the Mediterranean diet for kids makes sure they consume a healthy, balanced diet, form good eating habits, and get to eat a variety of tasty dishes that improve their general health and wellbeing.

1. Classic Greek Avgolemono Soup

Ingredients:

- 6 cups chicken broth

- ½ cup Arborio rice

- 2 eggs

- Juice of 2-3 lemons

- Cooked shredded chicken (optional)

- Salt and pepper to taste

- Fresh dill for garnish

Procedure:

1. Bring the chicken stock to a boil in a pot.

2. Cook the Arborio rice until it becomes soft.

3. Whisk eggs and lemon juice in a bowl until foamy.

4. Whisk continuously as you gradually add a ladle's worth of hot broth to the egg-lemon mixture.

5. Return the egg-lemon mixture to the pot gradually while continuing to whisk.

6. If desired, add some shredded chicken. Add pepper and salt for seasoning.

7. Simmer, without boiling, for a few minutes. Place some fresh dill on top.

Time Frame:

Preparation Time: 10 minutes

Cooking Time: 20 minutes

Total Time: 30 minutes

Yield:

Serves 4

Nutritional Value:

Average nutritional values per serving:

- Calories: 180 kcal

- Protein: 10g

- Carbohydrates: 20g

- Fat: 6g

- Fiber: 1g

Alternative Ingredients:

- Arborio rice can be substituted with orzo or another type of short pasta.

- Saffron can be substituted with turmeric for flavor and color.

2. Tuscan Tomato and Bread Soup (Pappa al Pomodoro)

Ingredients:

- 6 ripe tomatoes, chopped

- 4 cups vegetable broth

- 2 cups stale bread, diced

- 4 cloves garlic, minced

- 1 onion, chopped

- Fresh basil leaves

- Olive oil

- Salt and pepper to taste

- Grated Parmesan cheese (optional)

Procedure:

1. In a saucepan, sauté garlic and onion in olive oil until softened.

2. Add chopped tomatoes and cook until they break down.

3. Pour in the vegetable broth and bring to a simmer.

4. Add the stale bread and let it soak up the liquid.

5. Tear some basil leaves and stir them into the soup. Add pepper and salt for seasoning.

6. Simmer for 15-20 minutes until the bread is soft and the soup thickens.

7. Serve hot, garnished with fresh basil and grated Parmesan if desired.

Time Frame:

Preparation Time: 15 minutes

Cooking Time: 25 minutes

Total Time: 40 minutes

Yield:

Serves 6

Nutritional Value:

Average nutritional values per serving:

- Calories: 150 kcal

- Protein: 4g

- Carbohydrates: 25g

- Fat: 4g

- Fiber: 3g

Alternative Ingredients:

- Replace fresh tomatoes with canned crushed tomatoes.

- Use vegetable or chicken stock interchangeably.

3. Lentil and Vegetable Soup

Ingredients:

- 1 cup dried lentils, rinsed

- 4 cups vegetable broth

- 1 onion, diced

- 2 carrots, chopped

- 2 celery stalks, chopped

- 2 garlic cloves, minced

- 1 can diced tomatoes

- 1 teaspoon cumin

- 1 teaspoon paprika

- Salt and pepper to taste

- Fresh parsley for garnish

Procedure:

1. In a pot, combine lentils and vegetable broth. Bring to a boil, then reduce heat and simmer for 15 minutes.

2. Add diced onion, carrots, celery, and garlic. Cook for an additional 10 minutes.

3. Stir in diced tomatoes, cumin, paprika, salt, and pepper. Simmer for another 10-15 minutes until vegetables are tender.

4. Adjust seasoning as needed. Garnish with fresh parsley before serving.

Time Frame:

Preparation Time: 10 minutes

Cooking Time: 35-40 minutes

Total Time: 45-50 minutes

Yield:

Serves 4-6

Nutritional Value:

Average nutritional values per serving:

- Calories: 200 kcal

- Protein: 12g

- Carbohydrates: 35g

- Fat: 1g

- Fiber: 10g

Alternative Ingredients:

- Use any kind of lentil (red, green, or brown), depending on your taste.

- For variation, add other veggies like bell peppers or spinach.

4. Spanish Gazpacho

Ingredients:

- 6 ripe tomatoes, roughly chopped

- 1 cucumber, peeled and chopped

- 1 red bell pepper, seeded and chopped

- 2 cloves garlic, minced

- 1 small onion, chopped

- 1/4 cup olive oil

- 2 tablespoons red wine vinegar

- 2 cups tomato juice

- Salt and pepper to taste

- Fresh basil or cilantro for garnish

Procedure:

1. In a blender, combine tomatoes, cucumber, red bell pepper, garlic, onion, olive oil, and red wine vinegar. Process till smooth.

2. Pour the mixture into a bowl. Stir in tomato juice until desired consistency is obtained.

3. Add pepper and salt for seasoning. Refrigerate for at least 2 hours before serving.

4. Before serving cold, garnish with cilantro or fresh basil.

Time Frame:

Preparation Time: 15 minutes

Chilling Time: 2 hours

Total Time: 2 hours 15 minutes

Yield:

Serves 4-6

Nutritional Value:

Average nutritional values per serving:

- Calories: 120 kcal

- Protein: 2g

- Carbohydrates: 10g

- Fat: 8g

- Fiber: 2g

Alternative Ingredients:

- For a different tangy flavor, use sherry vinegar in place of red wine vinegar.

- Vary the amount of onion or garlic to suit your tastes.

5. Moroccan Chickpea Soup (Harira)

Ingredients:

- 1 cup dried chickpeas, soaked overnight

- 4 cups vegetable broth

- 1 onion, finely chopped

- 2 tomatoes, diced

- 2 tablespoons tomato paste

- 1/2 cup green lentils

- 2 tablespoons olive oil

- 1 teaspoon ground cumin

- 1 teaspoon ground ginger

- 1 teaspoon ground cinnamon

- Salt and pepper to taste

- Fresh cilantro for garnish

Procedure:

1. Soak the chickpeas and add the veggie broth to a saucepan. After bringing to a boil, simmer for thirty minutes.

2. Add the diced tomatoes, green lentils, chopped onion, ground cumin, ground ginger, ground cinnamon, olive oil, and salt and pepper. Cook until lentils and chickpeas are soft, about 20 to 25 minutes more.

3. Taste and adjust seasoning. Before serving, garnish with fresh cilantro.

Time Frame:

Preparation Time: 15 minutes (+ soaking time)

Cooking Time: 50-55 minutes

Total Time: Approximately 1 hour 10 minutes

Yield:

Serves 4-6

Nutritional Value:

Average nutritional values per serving:

- Calories: 250 kcal

- Protein: 10g

- Carbohydrates: 40g

- Fat: 6g

- Fiber: 10g

Alternative Ingredients:

When preparing, use canned chickpeas rather than dried ones to save time.

- Adapt ginger and cinnamon spices to your own tastes.

6. Italian Panzanella (Bread Salad)

Ingredients:

- 4 cups stale Italian bread, cubed

- 4 ripe tomatoes, chopped

- 1 cucumber, sliced

- 1 red onion, thinly sliced

- 1 bell pepper, diced

- 1/4 cup extra-virgin olive oil

- 2 tablespoons red wine vinegar

- Fresh basil leaves, torn

- Salt and pepper to taste

Procedure:

1. Mix the bell pepper, tomatoes, cucumber, red onion, and bread cubes in a bowl.

2. Over the mixture, drizzle some red wine vinegar and olive oil. To mix, toss.

3. Tumble in the basil leaves. Add pepper and salt for seasoning.

4. To allow the flavors to mingle, let the salad sit for 15 to 20 minutes before serving.

Time Frame:

Preparation Time: 15 minutes

Resting Time: 15-20 minutes

Total Time: 30-35 minutes

Yield:

Serves 4-6

Nutritional Value:

Average nutritional values per serving:

- Calories: 180 kcal

- Protein: 4g

- Carbohydrates: 25g

- Fat: 8g

- Fiber: 3g

Alternative Ingredients:

- You can use any rustic-textured bread, such ciabatta or sourdough.

- For added taste, add capers or olives.

7. Turkish Shepherd's Salad (Çoban Salatası)

Ingredients:

- 2 tomatoes, diced

- 1 cucumber, diced

- 1 red onion, finely chopped

- 1 green bell pepper, chopped

- 1/4 cup parsley, chopped

- 1/4 cup extra-virgin olive oil

- Juice of 1-2 lemons

- Salt and pepper to taste

Procedure:

1. Diced tomatoes, cucumber, bell pepper, red onion, and chopped parsley should all be combined in a bowl.

2. Over the salad, drizzle some lemon juice and olive oil. To coat, gently toss.

3. Adjust the amount of salt and pepper to taste.

4. Before serving, let it cool for fifteen to twenty minutes.

Time Frame:

Preparation Time: 10 minutes

Chilling Time: 15-20 minutes

Total Time: 25-30 minutes

Yield:

Serves 4-6

Nutritional Value:

Average nutritional values per serving:

- Calories: 120 kcal

- Protein: 2g

- Carbohydrates: 10g

- Fat: 8g

- Fiber: 3g

Alternative Ingredients:

- For a distinct tang, use red wine vinegar in instead of lemon juice.

To add even more freshness, add chopped mint leaves.

8. Grilled Vegetable Salad with Lemon-Herb Dressing

Ingredients:
- 2 zucchinis, sliced lengthwise
- 1 eggplant, sliced
- 1 red bell pepper, halved and seeded
- 1 yellow bell pepper, halved and seeded
- 1/4 cup olive oil
- Salt and pepper to taste
- Juice of 1 lemon
- 2 tablespoons chopped fresh herbs (basil, thyme, parsley)
- Mixed salad greens

Procedure:

1. Grill at a medium-high temperature. Apply a thin layer of olive oil to bell peppers, eggplants, and zucchini. Add pepper and salt for seasoning.

2. Vegetables should be grilled until soft and slightly browned. Take them off the burner and allow them cool.

3. Bite-sized chunks of grilled veggies should be added to a bowl.

4. Whisk together the chopped herbs, lemon juice, and leftover olive oil in a small bowl. After adding the dressing, gently toss the grilled vegetables.

5. Arrange the grilled veggies over a bed of mixed green salad leaves.

Time Frame:

Preparation Time: 15 minutes

Grilling Time: 10-15 minutes

Total Time: 25-30 minutes

Yield:

Serves 4-6

Nutritional Value:

Average nutritional values per serving:

- Calories: 150 kcal

- Protein: 2g

- Carbohydrates: 10g

- Fat: 12g

- Fiber: 4g

Alternative Ingredients:

- For the dressing, use any choice fresh herbs.

You are welcome to include or omit other grilled veggies, such as asparagus or mushrooms.

9. Tabbouleh (Lebanese Parsley Salad)

Ingredients:

- 1 cup bulgur wheat

- 1 1/2 cups boiling water

- 2 cups fresh parsley, finely chopped

- 1/2 cup fresh mint leaves, finely chopped

- 2 tomatoes, finely chopped

- 1 cucumber, finely chopped

- 1/4 cup red onion, finely chopped

- Juice of 2 lemons

- 1/4 cup extra-virgin olive oil

- Salt and pepper to taste

Procedure:

1. After placing bulgur wheat in a basin, cover it with boiling water. Once softened, cover and leave it for twenty to thirty minutes.

2. Using a fork, fluff the bulgur and allow it to come to room temperature.

3. Add the chopped parsley, mint, cucumber, tomatoes, and red onion to a large mixing bowl.

4. Mix thoroughly after adding the cold bulgur to the veggie bowl.

5. Whisk together lemon juice, olive oil, salt, and pepper in a small bowl. After adding the dressing to the salad, toss to mix.

6. To allow the flavors to mingle, refrigerate for at least an hour before serving.

Time Frame:

Preparation Time: 20 minutes (+ soaking time)

Resting Time: 1 hour

Total Time: Approximately 1 hour 20 minutes

Yield:

Serves 4-6

Nutritional Value:

Average nutritional values per serving:

- Calories: 180 kcal

- Protein: 4g

- Carbohydrates: 25g

- Fat: 8g

- Fiber: 6g

Alternative Ingredients:

- Use quinoa instead of bulgur for a gluten-free option.

- Adjust the ratio of parsley to mint based on personal taste preference.

10. Spanish Orange and Red Onion Salad (Ensalada de Naranja y Cebolla Roja)

Ingredients:

- 3-4 oranges, peeled and sliced

- 1 red onion, thinly sliced

- 2 tablespoons red wine vinegar

- 2 tablespoons extra-virgin olive oil

- Fresh parsley or cilantro for garnish

- Salt and pepper to taste

Procedure:

1. Place the orange slices in a plate for serving.

2. Arrange red onions in thin slices on top of the oranges.

3. To create the dressing, combine the olive oil, red wine vinegar, salt, and pepper in a small bowl.

4. Just before serving, drizzle the salad with the dressing.

5. Add some cilantro or parsley as a garnish.

Time Frame:

Preparation Time: 10 minutes

Total Time: 10 minutes

Yield:

Serves 4-6

Nutritional Value:

Average nutritional values per serving:

- Calories: 80 kcal

- Protein: 1g

- Carbohydrates: 10g

- Fat: 4g

- Fiber: 3g

Alternative Ingredients:

- For added taste, add some thinly sliced fennel or black olives.

- For a different flavor profile, try substituting balsamic vinegar or white wine vinegar.

1. Spanish Paella with Seafood

Ingredients:

- 2 cups bomba or Arborio rice

- 4 cups seafood or chicken broth

- 1 onion, chopped

- 4 cloves garlic, minced

- 1 red bell pepper, sliced

- 1 tomato, diced

- 1 teaspoon saffron threads

- 1 pound mixed seafood (shrimp, mussels, squid)

- 1/2 cup frozen peas

- 1 lemon, cut into wedges

- Salt and pepper to taste

- Olive oil

Procedure:

1. Heat the olive oil in a big skillet or paella pan over medium heat. Add the bell pepper, onion, and garlic and sauté until softened.

2. Cook the chopped tomato until it becomes soft.

3. Add rice and saffron threads and stir. For a few minutes, toast the rice.

4. Add the broth and heat until it boils. Simmer for approximately 15 minutes, uncovered, on low heat.

5. Over the rice, arrange a mixture of seafood. Put peas in. For ten to fifteen minutes, or until the seafood is cooked through, cook it covered.

6. Add pepper and salt for seasoning. Before serving, garnish with lemon wedges.

Time Frame:

Preparation Time: 15 minutes

Cooking Time: 30-35 minutes

Total Time: 45-50 minutes

Yield:

Serves 4-6

Nutritional Value:

Average nutritional values per serving:

- Calories: 350 kcal

- Protein: 20g

- Carbohydrates: 50g

- Fat: 6g

- Fiber: 3g

Alternative Ingredients:

- For modifications, try using chicken or veggies in place of seafood.

- To achieve a similar golden color, use turmeric instead of saffron.

2. Lebanese Rice Pilaf with Toasted Nuts

Ingredients:

- 2 cups basmati rice

- 4 cups chicken or vegetable broth

- 1 onion, finely chopped

- 1/2 cup mixed nuts (almonds, pine nuts)

- 2 tablespoons olive oil

- Salt and pepper to taste

- Fresh parsley for garnish

Procedure:

1. Till the water runs clear, rinse the basmati rice under cold water. Make sure to drain well.

2. Add the chopped onion to a pot with olive oil and sauté until transparent.

3. Stir the rice for a few minutes after adding it.

4. Add the broth and heat until it boils. Once the rice is done and the liquid has been absorbed, reduce heat, cover, and simmer for 15 to 20 minutes.

5. Toast the mixed nuts until they become gently brown in a different pan.

6. After the rice is done, use a fork to fluff it up. Add the roasted nuts and fold gently. Add pepper and salt for seasoning.

7. Before serving, garnish with fresh parsley.

Time Frame:

Preparation Time: 10 minutes

Cooking Time: 20-25 minutes

Total Time: 30-35 minutes

Yield:

Serves 4-6

Nutritional Value:

Average nutritional values per serving:

- Calories: 300 kcal

- Protein: 7g

- Carbohydrates: 50g

- Fat: 8g

- Fiber: 2g

Alternative Ingredients:

- Use a variety of nuts, such as cashews or pistachios.

- For a hint of sweetness, add raisins or dried apricots.

3. Greek Spanakorizo (Spinach and Rice)

Ingredients:

- 1 cup rice (preferably Arborio)

- 2 cups vegetable broth or water

- 1 onion, finely chopped

- 2 cloves garlic, minced

- 1 pound fresh spinach, chopped

- 1/4 cup chopped fresh dill

- Juice of 1 lemon

- Olive oil

- Salt and pepper to taste

Procedure:

1. Add the chopped onion and garlic to a pot and sauté in olive oil until transparent.

2. After adding, simmer the rice for a few minutes.

3. Add water or vegetable broth, then bring to a boil. Once the rice is cooked, reduce heat, cover, and simmer for 15 to 20 minutes.

4. After adding the chopped spinach, heat it until it wilts.

5. Add the lemon juice, salt, pepper, and chopped dill. Blend thoroughly.

6. Before serving, let it settle for a few minutes.

Time Frame:

Preparation Time: 10 minutes

Cooking Time: 25-30 minutes

Total Time: 35-40 minutes

Yield:

Serves 4-6

Nutritional Value:

Average nutritional values per serving:

- Calories: 180 kcal

- Protein: 5g

- Carbohydrates: 35g

- Fat: 2g

- Fiber: 4g

Alternative Ingredients:

- Use frozen spinach in place of fresh spinach.

- For variation, try using mint or parsley in place of or in addition to dill.

4. Italian Risotto with Asparagus and Parmesan

Ingredients:

- 1 1/2 cups Arborio rice

- 4 cups vegetable or chicken broth

- 1 onion, finely chopped

- 2 cloves garlic, minced

- 1 bunch asparagus, trimmed and chopped

- 1/2 cup grated Parmesan cheese

- 2 tablespoons butter

- Olive oil

- Salt and pepper to taste

Procedure:

1. Heat the broth in a pot over low heat.

2. Add the chopped onion and garlic to a separate skillet and sauté in olive oil until transparent.

3. After adding the Arborio rice, swirl it for a few minutes to coat it with oil.

4. One ladle at a time, gradually add heated broth to the rice, stirring constantly and letting the liquid soak in before adding more.

5. Add the chopped asparagus to another skillet and sauté until soft.

6. Add the butter, grated Parmesan cheese, salt, pepper, and sautéed asparagus to the creamy, al dente rice.

7. Before serving, let it a few minutes to rest.

Time Frame:

Preparation Time: 10 minutes

Cooking Time: 25-30 minutes

Total Time: 35-40 minutes

Yield:

Serves 4-6

Nutritional Value:

Average nutritional values per serving:

- Calories: 320 kcal

- Protein: 10g

- Carbohydrates: 50g

- Fat: 8g

- Fiber: 4g

Alternative Ingredients:

- Use peas or mushrooms in place of asparagus.

For a vegetarian variation, use vegetable broth.

5. Moroccan Couscous with Vegetables

Ingredients:

- 2 cups couscous

- 2 cups vegetable broth

- 2 tablespoons olive oil

- 1 onion, chopped

- 2 carrots, diced

- 1 zucchini, diced

- 1 red bell pepper, diced

- 1 teaspoon ground cumin

- 1 teaspoon ground coriander

- 1/2 teaspoon paprika

- Salt and pepper to taste

- Fresh cilantro for garnish

Procedure:

1. Bring the vegetable broth to a boil in a pot. Take off the heat and mix in the couscous. After covering, leave it for five minutes.

2. Using a fork, fluff the couscous and set it aside.

3. Saute chopped onion in olive oil in a pan until it becomes tender.

4. Add the red bell pepper, zucchini, and sliced carrots. Sauté the veggies until they are soft.

5. Add the paprika, ground cumin, ground coriander, salt, and pepper and stir.

6. Stir everything together in the pan after adding the cooked couscous.

7. Before serving, garnish with fresh cilantro.

Time Frame:

Preparation Time: 10 minutes

Cooking Time: 15-20 minutes

Total Time: 25-30 minutes

Yield:

Serves 4-6

Nutritional Value:

Average nutritional values per serving:

- Calories: 250 kcal

- Protein: 6g

- Carbohydrates: 45g

- Fat: 5g

- Fiber: 4g

Alternative Ingredients:

- Add additional veggies, such as squash or eggplant.

To provide more texture and taste, add raisins or chickpeas.

6. Turkish Bulgur Pilaf with Chickpeas

Ingredients:

- 1 cup bulgur wheat

- 2 cups vegetable broth

- 1 onion, finely chopped

- 2 cloves garlic, minced

- 1 can chickpeas, drained and rinsed

- 2 tablespoons olive oil

- Salt and pepper to taste

- Fresh parsley for garnish

Procedure:

1. After rinsing bulgur wheat in cold water, drain.

2. Add the chopped onion and garlic to a pan with olive oil and sauté until softened.

3. Cook the bulgur for a few minutes after adding it to the pan.

4. After adding the veggie broth, bring it to a boil. Simmer, covered, over low heat for 15 to 20 minutes, or until bulgur is soft and liquid is absorbed.

5. Add the chickpeas and stir. Add pepper and salt for seasoning.

6. Give it a few minutes to settle. Before serving, garnish with fresh parsley.

Time Frame:

Preparation Time: 10 minutes

Cooking Time: 20-25 minutes

Total Time: 30-35 minutes

Yield:

Serves 4-6

Nutritional Value:

Average nutritional values per serving:

- Calories: 200 kcal

- Protein: 7g

- Carbohydrates: 35g

- Fat: 4g

- Fiber: 8g

Alternative Ingredients:

- For variation, add chopped tomatoes or bell peppers.

- For a different texture, try using quinoa instead of bulgur.

7. Spanish Saffron Rice (Arroz con Azafrán)

Ingredients:

- 2 cups white rice

- 4 cups chicken broth

- Pinch of saffron threads

- 1 onion, finely chopped

- 2 cloves garlic, minced

- 1 red bell pepper, diced

- 2 tablespoons olive oil

- Salt to taste

Procedure:

1. Saffron threads should steep in 1/4 cup warm water in a small bowl for ten to fifteen minutes.

2. Add the chopped onion and garlic to a pan with olive oil and sauté until softened.

3. Cook the diced bell pepper for a few minutes after adding it.

4. After adding the rice to the pan, stir it for a few minutes.

5. Add the saffron water and chicken broth. Heat till boiling. Once the rice is done and the liquid has been absorbed, reduce heat, cover, and simmer for 15 to 20 minutes.

6. Reassembly rice with a fork. If necessary, season with salt right before serving.

Time Frame:

Preparation Time: 10 minutes

Cooking Time: 20-25 minutes

Total Time: 30-35 minutes

Yield:

Serves 4-6

Nutritional Value:

Average nutritional values per serving:

- Calories: 220 kcal

- Protein: 5g

- Carbohydrates: 45g

- Fat: 3g

- Fiber: 2g

Alternative Ingredients:

- For extra color and taste, add diced tomatoes, carrots, or peas.

- For a vegetarian alternative, use vegetable broth instead of chicken stock.

8. Greek Orzo Pasta with Lemon and Herbs

Ingredients:

- 1 cup orzo pasta

- 2 cups vegetable broth or water

- Zest and juice of 1 lemon

- 2 tablespoons olive oil

- 2 tablespoons chopped fresh herbs (such as parsley, dill, or oregano)

- Salt and pepper to taste

Procedure:

1. Bring water or vegetable broth to a boil in a pot.

2. Add the orzo pasta and cook it until al dente, following the directions on the package. After draining, set away.

3. Combine cooked orzo, olive oil, lemon zest, lemon juice, and finely chopped fresh herbs in a bowl.

4. Adjust the amount of salt and pepper to taste.

5. Heat or serve room temperature.

Time Frame:

Preparation Time: 5 minutes

Cooking Time: 10-12 minutes

Total Time: 15-17 minutes

Yield:

Serves 4-6

Nutritional Value:

Average nutritional values per serving:

- Calories: 180 kcal

- Protein: 4g

- Carbohydrates: 30g

- Fat: 5g

- Fiber: 2g

Alternative Ingredients:

- For additional taste and texture, add roasted veggies like bell peppers or cherry tomatoes.

- To create a different taste, try using various herbs like mint or basil.

9. Sicilian Rice Balls (Arancini)

Ingredients:

- 2 cups cooked risotto or Arborio rice

- 1 cup grated Parmesan cheese

- 1 cup breadcrumbs

- 1/2 cup mozzarella cheese, diced into small cubes

- 1/4 cup chopped fresh parsley

- 2 eggs, beaten

- Salt and pepper to taste

- Olive oil for frying

Procedure:

1. Cooked rice, beaten eggs, chopped parsley, breadcrumbs, grated Parmesan cheese, salt, and pepper should all be combined in a bowl.

2. Using your hand, flatten a tiny amount of the mixture and press a mozzarella cheese cube into the center. Gently form it into a ball, making sure the cheese stays inside.

3. In a pan over medium-high heat, warm the olive oil.

4. In batches, fry the rice balls until they are crispy and golden brown on all sides.

5. Take out of the oil and lay on a paper towel to absorb any leftover oil.

6. Serve hot as a tasty snack or appetizer.

Time Frame:

Preparation Time: 20 minutes

Cooking Time: 10-15 minutes (per batch)

Total Time: 30-35 minutes

Yield:

Makes approximately 12 arancini

Nutritional Value:

Average nutritional values per serving (1 arancino):

- Calories: 150 kcal

- Protein: 6g

- Carbohydrates: 18g

- Fat: 6g

- Fiber: 1g

Alternative Ingredients:

- For variation, stuff the rice balls with other contents, such as ground beef or peas.

- Make use of various cheeses, such as fontina or provolone.

10. Lebanese Freekeh with Chicken and Nuts

Ingredients:

- 1 cup freekeh, rinsed

- 2 cups chicken broth

- 1 onion, chopped

- 2 cloves garlic, minced

- 1 cup shredded cooked chicken

- 1/2 cup mixed nuts (such as almonds, pine nuts)

- 2 tablespoons olive oil

- Salt and pepper to taste

- Fresh mint for garnish

Procedure:

1. Add the chopped onion and garlic to a pot and sauté in olive oil until transparent.

2. After washing, add the freekeh and toast it for a few minutes.

3. Add the chicken broth and heat until it boils. Once the liquid has been absorbed and the freekeh is soft, reduce heat, cover, and simmer for 20 to 25 minutes.

4. Add mixed nuts and the shredded chicken and stir. Add pepper and salt for seasoning.

5. Give it a few minutes to settle. Before serving, garnish with fresh mint.

Time Frame:

Preparation Time: 10 minutes

Cooking Time: 25-30 minutes

Total Time: 35-40 minutes

Yield:

Serves 4-6

Nutritional Value:

Average nutritional values per serving:

- Calories: 280 kcal

- Protein: 15g

- Carbohydrates: 35g

- Fat: 10g

- Fiber: 8g

Alternative Ingredients:

- To get a distinct flavor profile, try using various nuts, such as walnuts or pistachios.

- For sweetness, add dried fruits like raisins or apricots.

1. Italian Spaghetti Aglio e Olio

Ingredients:

- 8 oz spaghetti

- 4 cloves garlic, thinly sliced

- 1/4 cup extra-virgin olive oil

- 1/2 teaspoon red pepper flakes (optional)

- Chopped fresh parsley for garnish

- Grated Parmesan cheese (optional)

- Salt to taste

Procedure:

1. Boil pasta in salted water until al dente, following the directions on the package. Before draining, save a cup of pasta water.

2. Warm up some olive oil in a pan over medium heat. Add the red pepper flakes (if using) and the sliced garlic. Sauté the garlic until it becomes yellow, but not burned.

3. In the pan, add the cooked spaghetti. Toss to ensure that the oil flavored with garlic coats the pasta evenly. To make a sauce, add some of the pasta water that was set aside if the pasta looks dry.

4. Use salt to season as desired.

5. Before serving, garnish with grated Parmesan cheese and chopped fresh parsley, if preferred.

Time Frame:

Preparation Time: 5 minutes

Cooking Time: 10-12 minutes

Total Time: 15-17 minutes

Yield:

Serves 2-3

Nutritional Value:

Average nutritional values per serving:

- Calories: 300 kcal

- Protein: 7g

- Carbohydrates: 45g

- Fat: 10g

- Fiber: 2g

Alternative Ingredients:

- Add sautéed shrimp or vegetables like broccoli or cherry tomatoes for variations.

2. Greek Pasta Salad with Mediterranean Vegetables

Ingredients:

- 8 oz pasta (penne, fusilli, or rotini)

- 1 cup cherry tomatoes, halved

- 1 cucumber, diced

- 1 bell pepper, diced

- 1/2 cup Kalamata olives, pitted and halved

- 1/4 cup red onion, thinly sliced

- 1/2 cup crumbled feta cheese

- 1/4 cup chopped fresh parsley

- 1/4 cup extra-virgin olive oil

- Juice of 1 lemon

- Salt and pepper to taste

Procedure:

1. Boil pasta in salted water according to package directions. After draining, rinse under cold water.

2. Cooked spaghetti, cherry tomatoes, cucumber, bell pepper, Kalamata olives, red onion, crumbled feta cheese, and chopped parsley should all be combined in a big bowl.

3. Over the salad, drizzle some lemon juice and olive oil. Gently toss to mix.

4. Adjust the amount of salt and pepper to taste.

5. Before serving, place in the refrigerator for at least one hour.

Time Frame:

Preparation Time: 15 minutes

Cooking Time: 10-12 minutes

Total Time: Approximately 25-27 minutes

Yield:

Serves 4-6

Nutritional Value:

Average nutritional values per serving:

- Calories: 280 kcal

- Protein: 8g

- Carbohydrates: 35g

- Fat: 12g

- Fiber: 3g

Alternative Ingredients:

- For extra taste, add roasted red peppers or artichoke hearts.

- If you have dietary restrictions, use whole wheat or gluten-free pasta.

3. Moroccan Lamb and Vegetable Couscous

Ingredients:

- 1 lb lamb, diced

- 1 cup couscous

- 2 cups chicken or vegetable broth

- 1 onion, chopped

- 2 carrots, sliced

- 1 zucchini, diced

- 1 can chickpeas, drained and rinsed

- 2 tomatoes, diced

- 2 tablespoons olive oil

- 2 teaspoons ground cumin

- 2 teaspoons ground coriander

- 1 teaspoon paprika

- Salt and pepper to taste

- Chopped fresh cilantro for garnish

Procedure:

1. Warm up the olive oil in a pot over medium heat. Cut onion and sauté till tender.

2. Cook the diced lamb until it turns golden.

3. Add the paprika, ground cumin, ground coriander, salt, and pepper and stir.

4. Add the chickpeas, tomatoes, zucchini, and carrots. Simmer for a short while.

5. Add the vegetable or chicken broth and heat until it boils. Once the vegetables are soft, reduce the heat and simmer for ten to fifteen minutes.

6. Boil two cups of water in a different pot. Take off the heat, stir in the couscous, cover, and let for five minutes. Coat the couscous in a fork.

7. Over the cooked couscous, serve the stew of lamb and vegetables.

8. Before serving, add some freshly cut cilantro as a garnish.

Time Frame:

Preparation Time: 15 minutes

Cooking Time: 25-30 minutes

Total Time: 40-45 minutes

Yield:

Serves 4-6

Nutritional Value:

Average nutritional values per serving:

- Calories: 380 kcal

- Protein: 25g

- Carbohydrates: 40g

- Fat: 14g

- Fiber: 6g

Alternative Ingredients:

- Instead of using lamb, use beef or chicken.

- To add a little sweetness, add raisins or apricots.

4. Sicilian Pasta alla Norma

Ingredients:

- 8 oz pasta (rigatoni or spaghetti)

- 2 cups tomato sauce

- 2 eggplants, diced

- 3 cloves garlic, minced

- 1/2 cup grated ricotta salata or Parmesan cheese

- Fresh basil leaves for garnish

- Olive oil

- Salt and pepper to taste

Procedure:

1. Turn the oven on to 400°F, or 200°C. Diced eggplant should be put on a baking pan, covered with olive oil, and baked for 20 to 25 minutes, or until soft and browned.

2. Boil pasta in salted water until al dente, following the directions on the package. After draining, set away.

3. Warm up some olive oil in a pan over medium heat. Garlic, minced, and sauté until aromatic.

4. Add the tomato sauce and boil for a while.

5. To the sauce, add the roasted eggplant. Simmer for a few minutes to let the flavors meld.

6. Mix the sauce with the cooked pasta.

7. Serve hot, topped with fresh basil leaves and grated Parmesan or ricotta salata cheese.

Time Frame:

Preparation Time: 15 minutes

Cooking Time: 25-30 minutes

Total Time: Approximately 40-45 minutes

Yield:

Serves 2-3

Nutritional Value:

Average nutritional values per serving:

- Calories: 320 kcal

- Protein: 10g

- Carbohydrates: 50g

- Fat: 8g

- Fiber: 6g

Alternative Ingredients:

- Instead of using ricotta salata, use fresh mozzarella or goat cheese.

- For a spicy kick, add a little pinch of red pepper flakes.

5. Turkish Manti (Mini Dumplings in Yogurt Sauce)

Ingredients:

For the Dough:

- 2 cups all-purpose flour

- 1/2 cup water

- 1 egg

- Salt to taste

For the Filling:

- 1/2 lb ground beef or lamb

- 1 onion, finely chopped

- 1/2 teaspoon ground cumin

- 1/2 teaspoon paprika

- Salt and pepper to taste

For the Yogurt Sauce:

- 2 cups plain yogurt

- 2 cloves garlic, minced

- 2 tablespoons olive oil

- Salt to taste

Procedure:

Making the Dough:

1. Mix the flour, egg, water, and salt together in a bowl. Work the dough until it becomes smooth. After 30 minutes, cover and let it rest.

Making the Filling:

2. Combine the ground meat, chopped onion, paprika, ground cumin, and salt and pepper in a separate bowl.

Assembly:

3. Cut the dough into small squares after rolling it out thinly.

4. Put a tiny bit of filling in the middle of every square. To create small parcels, fold the corners (like tortellini).

Cooking:

5. The dumplings should float to the top after 10 to 12 minutes of boiling in salted water.

Making the Yogurt Sauce:

6. Combine yogurt, salt, and minced garlic in another bowl.

7. In a skillet with heated olive oil, sauté some dried mint until fragrant.

8. Over the yogurt sauce, drizzle the oil scented with mint.

Serve the fried manti with mint oil and yogurt sauce on top.

Time Frame:

Preparation Time: 45 minutes

Cooking Time: 10-12 minutes

Total Time: Approximately 55-57 minutes

Yield:

Serves 4-6

Nutritional Value:

Average nutritional values per serving:

- Calories: 300 kcal

- Protein: 15g

- Carbohydrates: 30g

- Fat: 14g

- Fiber: 2g

Alternative Ingredients:

- For a vegetarian version, use ground chicken or tofu.

- To enhance the flavor of the yogurt sauce, add tomato sauce or chili flakes.

6. Spanish Seafood Paella Pasta

Ingredients:

- 8 oz spaghetti or linguine

- 1 lb mixed seafood (shrimp, mussels, squid)

- 1 onion, diced

- 2 cloves garlic, minced

- 1 red bell pepper, diced

- 1 tomato, diced

- 1 teaspoon smoked paprika

- 1 teaspoon saffron threads

- 2 cups chicken or seafood broth

- 2 tablespoons olive oil

- Salt and pepper to taste

- Chopped fresh parsley for garnish

Procedure:

1. Boil pasta in salted water according to package directions. After draining, set away.

2. Heat the olive oil in a big skillet or paella pan over medium heat. Cut onion and sauté till tender.

3. Add the diced red bell pepper and minced garlic. Simmer for a short while.

4. Put a variety of seafood on the pan. Cook until the edges begin to get opaque.

5. Add the saffron threads, diced tomato, smoked paprika, salt, and pepper and stir.

6. Add the broth made from chicken or fish, then simmer. Cook it for five to seven minutes.

7. Cooked pasta should be added to the skillet and mixed with the sauce and seafood.

8. Before serving, sprinkle some freshly chopped parsley on top.

Time Frame:

Preparation Time: 15 minutes

Cooking Time: 15-20 minutes

Total Time: Approximately 30-35 minutes

Yield:

Serves 2-3

Nutritional Value:

Average nutritional values per serving:

- Calories: 350 kcal

- Protein: 25g

- Carbohydrates: 40g

- Fat: 10g

- Fiber: 3g

Alternative Ingredients:

- To get varied flavors, try using different kinds of shellfish or switching it up with chicken or chorizo.

- For added texture, add peas or artichoke hearts.

7. Lebanese Kibbeh (Bulgur and Minced Meat)

Ingredients:

For the Kibbeh Shell:

- 1 cup fine bulgur wheat

- 1 lb ground beef or lamb

- 1 onion, finely chopped

- 1 teaspoon ground allspice

- 1 teaspoon ground cinnamon

- Salt and pepper to taste

- Olive oil for greasing

For the Filling:

- 1/2 lb ground beef or lamb

- 1 onion, finely chopped

- 2 tablespoons pine nuts

- 1/2 teaspoon ground cinnamon

- Salt and pepper to taste

- Olive oil for cooking

Procedure:

Preparing the Kibbeh Shell:

1. After soaking bulgur wheat in water for ten to fifteen minutes, remove any extra water.

2. Combine bulgur, chopped onion, ground cinnamon, ground allspice, and salt and pepper. Work the mixture into the consistency of dough.

3. Spread some olive oil on a baking dish. To construct the base, evenly press half of the bulgur and meat mixture into the dish's bottom.

Making the Filling:

4. Warm up some olive oil in a pan over medium heat. Chop the onion and sauté it until transparent.

5. Cook the ground meat until it turns brown.

6. Add the ground cinnamon, pine nuts, salt, and pepper and stir. Simmer for a few minutes to let the flavors meld.

Assembly:

7. Cover the bottom layer of the baking dish with the prepared filling.

8. Gently press the leftover bulgur and meat mixture between two pieces of wax paper. Gently press it to seal the edges as you carefully arrange it over the filling.

Baking:

9. Set oven temperature to 175°C/350°F. Bake the kibbeh for thirty to forty minutes, or until the top is browned.

Time Frame:

Preparation Time: 30 minutes

Cooking Time: 30-40 minutes

Total Time: Approximately 60-70 minutes

Yield:

Serves 4-6

Nutritional Value:

Average nutritional values per serving:

- Calories: 320 kcal

- Protein: 25g

- Carbohydrates: 20g

- Fat: 15g

- Fiber: 3g

Alternative Ingredients:

- To make it leaner, use ground turkey or chicken.

- Chopped almonds or walnuts can be used in place of pine nuts.

8. Italian Fettuccine Alfredo with Spinach and Cherry Tomatoes

Ingredients:

- 8 oz fettuccine pasta

- 1 cup heavy cream

- 1/2 cup grated Parmesan cheese

- 2 cups fresh spinach leaves

- 1 cup cherry tomatoes, halved

- 2 cloves garlic, minced

- 2 tablespoons butter

- Salt and pepper to taste

- Chopped fresh basil for garnish

Procedure:

1. Boil salted water and cook fettuccine pasta as directed on the package. After draining, set away.

2. Melt butter in a pan over a medium heat. Garlic, minced, and sauté until aromatic.

3. After adding the heavy cream, boil the mixture. Give it a minute or two to cook.

4. When the sauce thickens, whisk in the grated Parmesan cheese.

5. Add the cherry tomatoes cut in half and the fresh spinach leaves. Simmer until the tomatoes are tender and the spinach wilts.

6. When the fettuccine is cooked, add it to the sauce and toss to coat it evenly.

7. Adjust the amount of salt and pepper to taste.

8. Before serving, garnish with finely chopped fresh basil.

Time Frame:

Preparation Time: 10 minutes

Cooking Time: 15-20 minutes

Total Time: Approximately 25-30 minutes

Yield:

Serves 2-3

Nutritional Value:

Average nutritional values per serving:

- Calories: 450 kcal

- Protein: 12g

- Carbohydrates: 40g

- Fat: 28g

- Fiber: 3g

Alternative Ingredients:

- If you have dietary restrictions, use whole wheat or gluten-free pasta.

- Use kale or arugula in place of spinach.

9. Greek Pastitsio (Baked Pasta with Meat Sauce)

Ingredients:

For the Meat Sauce:

- 1 lb ground beef or lamb

- 1 onion, chopped

- 2 cloves garlic, minced

- 1 can crushed tomatoes

- 2 tablespoons tomato paste

- 1 teaspoon ground cinnamon

- 1 teaspoon dried oregano

- Salt and pepper to taste

- Olive oil for cooking

For the Pasta and Topping:

- 8 oz penne or macaroni pasta

- 1/2 cup grated Parmesan cheese

- 2 cups béchamel sauce (white sauce)

- 1/4 cup breadcrumbs

- Butter for greasing

Procedure:

Making the Meat Sauce:

1. Warm up some olive oil in a pan over medium heat. Chop the onion and sauté it until transparent.

2. Add the ground beef and minced garlic. Cook the meat until it takes on color.

3. Add the tomato paste, ground cinnamon, dried oregano, smashed tomatoes, salt, and pepper and stir. Simmer until the sauce thickens, about 15 to 20 minutes.

Preparing the Pasta and Assembly:

4. Boil pasta in salted water according to package directions. After draining, set away.

5. Set oven temperature to 175°C/350°F. Spread butter to coat the bottom of a baking dish, then scatter breadcrumbs on top.

6. Arrange the cooked spaghetti half-way across the breadcrumbs.

7. Cover the spaghetti layer with half of the meat sauce.

8. Evenly cover the beef sauce with half of the béchamel sauce.

9. With the remaining spaghetti, meat sauce, and béchamel sauce, repeat the layering.

10. Top with grated Parmesan cheese.

Baking:

11. Bake for 40 to 45 minutes, or until the top is golden brown, in a preheated oven.

12. Before serving, let it cool for a few minutes.

Time Frame:

Preparation Time: 30 minutes

Cooking Time: 1 hour

Total Time: Approximately 1 hour 30 minutes

Yield:

Serves 6-8

Nutritional Value:

Average nutritional values per serving:

- Calories: 480 kcal

- Protein: 25g

- Carbohydrates: 40g

- Fat: 25g

- Fiber: 3g

Alternative Ingredients:

- Use ground chicken or turkey as a leaner **Alternative** to beef or lamb.

- Replace béchamel sauce with a mixture of Greek yogurt and eggs for a lighter option.

Ingredients:

For the Chicken Tagine:

- 4 chicken thighs (bone-in, skin-on)

- 1 onion, chopped

- 2 cloves garlic, minced

- 1 teaspoon ground cumin

- 1 teaspoon ground ginger

- 1 teaspoon ground turmeric

- 1 teaspoon paprika

- 1 cinnamon stick

- 1 cup chicken broth

- 1 cup canned chickpeas, drained and rinsed

- 1 cup chopped tomatoes

- 1/2 cup dried apricots, chopped

- 2 tablespoons olive oil

- Salt and pepper to taste

- Fresh cilantro for garnish

For the Couscous:

- 1 cup couscous

- 1 1/2 cups chicken broth or water

- 1 tablespoon butter

- Salt to taste

Procedure:

Preparing the Chicken Tagine:

1. Salt, pepper, ground cumin, ground ginger, ground turmeric, and paprika are used to season chicken thighs.

2. Heat the olive oil in a big skillet or tagine over medium-high heat. Chicken thighs should be seared until all sides are golden brown. Take out and place aside.

3. Minced garlic and chopped onion should be sautéed in the same pan until they are tender.

4. Put the pan back where the cooked chicken thighs were. Add the dried apricots, cinnamon stick, canned chickpeas, diced tomatoes, and chicken broth.

5. Once the chicken is soft and cooked through, boil it covered for 25 to 30 minutes.

Making the Couscous:

6. Bring water or chicken broth to a boil in a different pot. Add salt and butter.

7. After adding the couscous, cover and take the pot off the stove. Give it five minutes to sit. Using a fork, fluff the couscous.

Serving:

8. Over the cooked couscous, serve the Moroccan Chicken Tagine.

9. Before serving, garnish with fresh cilantro.

Time Frame:

Preparation Time: 20 minutes

Cooking Time: 30-35 minutes

Total Time: Approximately 50-55 minutes

Yield:

Serves 4

Nutritional Value:

Average nutritional values per serving:

- Calories: 420 kcal

- Protein: 25g

- Carbohydrates: 35g

- Fat: 20g

- Fiber: 5g

Alternative Ingredients:

- Use chicken drumsticks or breasts in place of chicken thighs.

- For a different sweetness, try substituting raisins or prunes for the dried apricots.

1. Spanish Fabada Asturiana (Bean Stew)

Ingredients:

- 1 lb dried white beans (Asturian faba beans if available)

- 4 chorizo sausages, sliced

- 1 lb pork shoulder or bacon, diced

- 1 onion, chopped

- 3 cloves garlic, minced

- 2 bay leaves

- 1 teaspoon sweet paprika

- 6 cups chicken broth or water

- Salt and pepper to taste

- Olive oil

Procedure:

1. For one night, soak the dried beans in water.

2. Heat the olive oil in a big pot or Dutch oven over medium heat. Minced garlic and diced onion should be sautéed until transparent.

3. Add the sliced chorizo and the diced pork shoulder (or bacon). Sauté till browned.

4. Add the bay leaves, sweet paprika, soaking beans, salt, and pepper and stir.

5. Add water or chicken broth. After bringing to a boil, turn down the heat. Simmer for two to three hours, or until the stew thickens and the beans are soft.

6. Before serving, take off the bay leaves.

Time Frame:

Preparation Time: 15 minutes (+ overnight soaking)

Cooking Time: 2-3 hours

Total Time: Approximately 3 hours 15 minutes

Yield:

Serves 6-8

Nutritional Value:

Average nutritional values per serving:

- Calories: 380 kcal

- Protein: 25g

- Carbohydrates: 35g

- Fat: 15g

- Fiber: 10g

Alternative Ingredients:

- Use smoked paprika for a deeper flavor.

- Substitute pork with chicken or omit for a vegetarian version.

2. Greek Fasolada (Bean Soup)

Ingredients:

- 1 cup dried white beans (Great Northern beans)

- 1 onion, chopped

- 2 carrots, diced

- 2 celery stalks, chopped

- 2 cloves garlic, minced

- 2 bay leaves

- 1 can chopped tomatoes

- 4 cups vegetable or chicken broth

- 2 tablespoons olive oil

- Salt and pepper to taste

- Chopped fresh parsley for garnish

Procedure:

1. Soak dry beans for several hours or perhaps overnight in water.

2. Warm up the olive oil in a pot over medium heat. Add the minced garlic, diced onion, carrots, and celery and sauté until softened.

3. Stir in the soaked beans, bay leaves, chopped tomatoes from a can, chicken or veggie broth, salt, and pepper.

4. Once the beans are soft, reduce the heat and simmer for one and a half to two hours.

5. Taste and adjust seasoning.

6. Garnish with freshly cut parsley and serve hot.

Time Frame:

Preparation Time: 15 minutes (+ soaking time)

Cooking Time: 1.5-2 hours

Total Time: Approximately 2 hours 15 minutes

Yield:

Serves 4-6

Nutritional Value:

Average nutritional values per serving:

- Calories: 240 kcal

- Protein: 12g

- Carbohydrates: 40g

- Fat: 5g

- Fiber: 10g

Alternative Ingredients:

- To add a tart twist, squeeze in some lemon juice.

- Add chopped kale or spinach for extra nutrition.

Ingredients:

- 1 cup small pasta (like ditalini or elbow macaroni)

- 1 can cannellini beans, drained and rinsed

- 1 onion, chopped

- 2 cloves garlic, minced

- 1 carrot, diced

- 1 celery stalk, diced

- 1 can crushed tomatoes

- 4 cups vegetable or chicken broth

- 2 tablespoons olive oil

- 1 teaspoon dried oregano

- Salt and pepper to taste

- Grated Parmesan cheese for garnish

Procedure:

1. Boil pasta in salted water according to package directions. After draining, set away.

2. Warm up the olive oil in a pot over medium heat. Diced carrot, diced celery, minced garlic, and chopped onion should all be sautéed until soft.

3. Add the dried oregano, crushed tomatoes from cans, cannellini beans, vegetable or chicken broth, salt, and pepper.

4. Simmer 15 to 20 minutes to let the flavors combine.

5. Just before serving, stir in cooked pasta.

6. Garnish with grated Parmesan cheese and serve hot.

Time Frame:

Preparation Time: 15 minutes

Cooking Time: 20-25 minutes

Total Time: Approximately 40 minutes

Yield:

Serves 4-6

Nutritional Value:

Average nutritional values per serving:

- Calories: 280 kcal

- Protein: 10g

- Carbohydrates: 45g

- Fat: 6g

- Fiber: 8g

Alternative Ingredients:

- Use different kinds of beans, such as navy or red kidney beans.

- For a hint of heat, add a sprinkle of red pepper flakes.

4. Turkish Red Lentil Köfte

Ingredients:

- 1 cup red lentils

- 1 onion, finely chopped

- 2 tablespoons tomato paste

- 1/2 cup fine bulgur

- 1 teaspoon ground cumin

- 1 teaspoon paprika

- 1 teaspoon dried mint

- Salt and pepper to taste

- Olive oil for frying

Procedure:

1. Boil the red lentils until they become tender. After removing any extra water, allow them to cool somewhat.

2. Cooked red lentils, chopped onion, tomato paste, fine bulgur, paprika, ground cumin, dried mint, salt, and pepper should all be combined in a bowl. Blend until thoroughly blended.

3. Form the mixture into tiny köfte, either oval or ball shaped.

4. In a pan set over medium heat, warm the olive oil. Cook köfte until both sides are golden brown.

5. Köfte can be served warm or cold.

Time Frame:

Preparation Time: 15 minutes (+ cooling time)

Cooking Time: 15-20 minutes

Total Time: Approximately 35 minutes

Yield:

Makes about 12 köfte

Nutritional Value:

Average nutritional values per serving (2 köfte):

- Calories: 200 kcal

- Protein: 8g

- Carbohydrates: 35g

- Fat: 2g

- Fiber: 8g

Alternative Ingredients:

- For more taste, try adding other spices like sumac or chili flakes.

- Incorporate finely chopped fresh cilantro or parsley into the mixture.

5. Moroccan Chickpea and Vegetable Tagine

Ingredients:

- 2 cups cooked chickpeas

- 1 onion, chopped

- 2 carrots, sliced

- 1 zucchini, diced

- 1 eggplant, diced

- 2 cloves garlic, minced

- 1 can chopped tomatoes

- 1 teaspoon ground cumin

- 1 teaspoon ground coriander

- 1 teaspoon paprika

- Pinch of saffron threads (optional)

- Salt and pepper to taste

- Olive oil

- Fresh cilantro for garnish

Procedure:

1. Heat the olive oil in a big skillet or tagine over medium heat. Minced garlic and diced onion should be sautéed till tender.

2. Add the diced eggplant, zucchini, and carrots. Simmer for a short while.

3. Add the paprika, ground coriander, ground cumin, and saffron threads (if using).

4. Add salt, pepper, canned chopped tomatoes, and cooked chickpeas. Vegetables should simmer for 20 to 25 minutes to become soft.

5. Taste and adjust seasoning.

6. Before serving, garnish with fresh cilantro.

Time Frame:

Preparation Time: 15 minutes (+ chickpea cooking time)

Cooking Time: 25-30 minutes

Total Time: Approximately 40-45 minutes

Yield:

Serves 4-6

Nutritional Value:

Average nutritional values per serving:

- Calories: 220 kcal

- Protein: 8g

- Carbohydrates: 35g

- Fat: 5g

- Fiber: 10g

Alternative Ingredients:

- Add additional veggies, such as potatoes or bell peppers.

- Squeeze in some lemon juice for added freshness.

6. Spanish Garlic White Bean Soup (Sopa de Ajo)

Ingredients:

- 2 cans white beans (cannellini or navy beans), drained and rinsed

- 6 cups vegetable or chicken broth

- 6 cloves garlic, minced

- 2 teaspoons smoked paprika

- 1 teaspoon ground cumin

- 2 tablespoons olive oil

- Salt and pepper to taste

- Chopped fresh parsley for garnish

Procedure:

1. Warm up the olive oil in a pot over medium heat. Garlic, minced, and sauté until aromatic.

2. Add the ground cumin, smoked paprika, drained white beans, salt, and pepper. Simmer for a short while.

3. Add the chicken or veggie broth. To blend flavors, bring to a simmer and cook for 15 to 20 minutes.

4. Using a hand blender or a normal blender, mix some of the soup until it becomes creamy.

5. Stir thoroughly and add back the blended portion to the pot.

6. Taste and adjust seasoning.

7. Garnish with freshly cut parsley and serve hot.

Time Frame:

Preparation Time: 10 minutes

Cooking Time: 20-25 minutes

Total Time: Approximately 30-35 minutes

Yield:

Serves 4-6

Nutritional Value:

Average nutritional values per serving:

- Calories: 180 kcal

- Protein: 8g

- Carbohydrates: 25g

- Fat: 5g

- Fiber: 7g

Alternative Ingredients:

- For a little kick of spice, add a sprinkle of crushed red pepper flakes.

- Before serving, pour some extra virgin olive oil on top for flavor.

7. Lebanese Mujadara (Lentils and Rice)

Ingredients:

- 1 cup brown or green lentils, rinsed

- 1 cup basmati rice

- 2 onions, thinly sliced

- 4 cups vegetable or chicken broth

- 2 tablespoons olive oil

- 1 teaspoon ground cumin

- 1 teaspoon ground coriander

- Salt and pepper to taste

- Chopped fresh parsley or cilantro for garnish

Procedure:

1. Warm up the olive oil in a pot over medium heat. Onions cut thinly should be sautéed until crispy and caramelized. Take out and place aside.

2. To the pot, add the washed lentils, basmati rice, ground coriander, ground cumin, and salt and pepper. Simmer for a short while.

3. Add the chicken or veggie broth. After bringing to a boil, lower the heat to low, cover, and simmer for 20 to 25 minutes, or until the rice and lentils are soft and the liquid has been absorbed.

4. Top the jamadara with chopped fresh cilantro or parsley and caramelized onions.

Time Frame:

Preparation Time: 10 minutes

Cooking Time: 25-30 minutes

Total Time: Approximately 35-40 minutes

Yield:

Serves 4-6

Nutritional Value:

Average nutritional values per serving:

- Calories: 280 kcal

- Protein: 10g

- Carbohydrates: 50g

- Fat: 5g

- Fiber: 8g

Alternative Ingredients:

- For a nuttier flavor, replace basmati rice with brown rice.

- For a faint flavor boost, mix with a small pinch of ground cinnamon.

8. Italian Cannellini Bean Salad with Herbs

Ingredients:

- 2 cans cannellini beans, drained and rinsed

- 1 red onion, finely chopped

- 2 tablespoons fresh parsley, chopped

- 2 tablespoons fresh basil, chopped

- 2 tablespoons fresh oregano, chopped

- 3 tablespoons extra virgin olive oil

- 2 tablespoons red wine vinegar

- Salt and pepper to taste

Procedure:

1. Fresh herbs (parsley, basil, and oregano) and finely chopped red onion go well with drained and rinsed cannellini beans in a bowl.

2. Over the bean mixture, drizzle with extra virgin olive oil and red wine vinegar.

3. Adjust the amount of salt and pepper to taste.

4. Gently toss until all items are thoroughly mixed.

5. Before serving, let the flavors mingle for at least 15 to 20 minutes.

Time Frame:

Preparation Time: 10 minutes

Total Time: Approximately 10 minutes (plus resting time)

Yield:

Serves 4-6

Nutritional Value:

Average nutritional values per serving:

- Calories: 200 kcal

- Protein: 9g

- Carbohydrates: 25g

- Fat: 8g

- Fiber: 7g

Alternative Ingredients:

- For a distinct tang, try substituting balsamic vinegar for red wine vinegar.

- For added freshness, cut some cucumber or cherry tomatoes.

9. Greek Gigantes Plaki (Baked Giant Beans)

Ingredients:

- 2 cans gigantes beans (large white beans), drained and rinsed

- 1 onion, finely chopped

- 2 cloves garlic, minced

- 1 can chopped tomatoes

- 1/4 cup chopped fresh parsley

- 2 tablespoons tomato paste

- 1 teaspoon dried oregano

- 1 teaspoon paprika

- 1/4 cup extra virgin olive oil

- Salt and pepper to taste

Procedure:

1. Set oven temperature to 175°C/350°F.

2. Drained gigantes beans, minced garlic, finely chopped onion, chopped tomatoes, chopped fresh parsley, tomato paste, dried oregano, paprika, extra virgin olive oil, salt, and pepper should all be combined in a baking dish.

3. To make sure all the ingredients are dispersed evenly, thoroughly mix.

4. Bake the baking dish for 40 to 45 minutes while covered with foil.

5. After removing the foil, bake for a further 10 to 15 minutes, or until the top begins to turn brown.

6. Serve heated Gigantes Plaki.

Time Frame:

Preparation Time: 15 minutes

Cooking Time: 55-60 minutes

Total Time: Approximately 1 hour 15 minutes

Yield:

Serves 4-6

Nutritional Value:

Average nutritional values per serving:

- Calories: 280 kcal

- Protein: 9g

- Carbohydrates: 35g

- Fat: 12g

- Fiber: 10g

Alternative Ingredients:

- Chopped fresh mint or dill can be added for an additional herbal taste.

- Add a squeeze of lemon juice for a zesty variation.

10. Moroccan Harira (Chickpea and Lentil Soup)

Ingredients:

- 1 cup dried chickpeas, soaked overnight

- 1/2 cup dried lentils

- 1 onion, chopped

- 2 stalks celery, chopped

- 2 carrots, diced

- 3 cloves garlic, minced

- 1 can diced tomatoes

- 6 cups vegetable or chicken broth

- 2 tablespoons tomato paste

- 2 teaspoons ground cumin

- 1 teaspoon ground ginger

- 1 teaspoon paprika

- Pinch of saffron threads (optional)

- Salt and pepper to taste

- Olive oil

- Chopped fresh cilantro for garnish

Procedure:

1. Warm up the olive oil in a pot over medium heat. Diced carrots, celery, minced garlic, and chopped onion should all be sautéed until soft.

2. Add the dried lentils, diced tomatoes, paprika, ground cumin, ground ginger, drained and soaked chickpeas, tomato paste, saffron threads (if using), salt, and pepper.

3. After bringing to a boil, turn down the heat. Cook, covered, until lentils and chickpeas are soft, about 1 to 2 hours.

4. Taste and adjust seasoning.

5. Garnish with freshly cut cilantro and serve hot.

Time Frame:

Preparation Time: 15 minutes (+ soaking time)

Cooking Time: 1.5-2 hours

Total Time: Approximately 2 hours 15 minutes

Yield:

Serves 6-8

Nutritional Value:

Average nutritional values per serving:

- Calories: 240 kcal

- Protein: 10g

- Carbohydrates: 35g

- Fat: 6g

- Fiber: 10g

Alternative Ingredients:

- To add flavor and scent, add a pinch of cinnamon.

- Add chopped kale or spinach for additional greens.

1. Italian Caponata (Eggplant Stew)

Ingredients:

- 2 large eggplants, diced

- 2 tablespoons olive oil

- 1 onion, finely chopped

- 2 cloves garlic, minced

- 1 can diced tomatoes

- 2 tablespoons red wine vinegar

- 2 tablespoons capers, drained

- 1/4 cup chopped green olives

- 2 tablespoons sugar

- Salt and pepper to taste

- Chopped fresh basil for garnish

Procedure:

1. In a pan set over medium heat, warm the olive oil. Diced eggplant should be sautéed till golden brown. Take out and place aside.

2. If necessary, add a little extra oil to the same pan. Minced garlic and diced onion should be sautéed till tender.

3. Add the chopped green olives, red wine vinegar, capers, diced tomatoes, sugar, salt, and pepper.

4. Simmer for a few minutes to gently thicken the sauce.

5. Return the cooked eggplants to the pan. Simmer for ten to fifteen minutes.

6. Before serving, garnish with finely chopped fresh basil.

Time Frame:

Preparation Time: 15 minutes

Cooking Time: 25-30 minutes

Total Time: Approximately 40-45 minutes

Yield:

Serves 4-6

Nutritional Value:

Average nutritional values per serving:

- Calories: 150 kcal

- Protein: 2g

- Carbohydrates: 20g

- Fat: 8g

- Fiber: 6g

Alternative Ingredients:

- For more texture and richness, add almonds or pine nuts.

If preferred, replace the green olives with black olives.

2. Greek Briam (Roasted Vegetables)

Ingredients:

- 2 large potatoes, sliced

- 2 zucchinis, sliced

- 2 eggplants, sliced

- 2 bell peppers (red and green), sliced

- 4 tomatoes, sliced

- 1 onion, thinly sliced

- 4 cloves garlic, minced

- 1/4 cup olive oil

- 2 tablespoons chopped fresh parsley

- 1 tablespoon chopped fresh oregano (or 1 teaspoon dried oregano)

- Salt and pepper to taste

Procedure:

1. Turn the oven on to 375°F, or 190°C.

2. Sliced potatoes, zucchini, eggplants, bell peppers, tomatoes, thinly sliced onion, minced garlic, olive oil, chopped fresh oregano, chopped fresh parsley, salt, and pepper should all be well coated after being combined in a big bowl.

3. Evenly distribute the veggie mixture into a baking dish.

4. Bake the dish for 45 to 50 minutes with foil covering it.

5. After removing the foil, bake the vegetables for a further 15 to 20 minutes, or until they are soft and starting to brown.

6. Warm Briam should be served.

Time Frame:

Preparation Time: 20 minutes

Cooking Time: 60-70 minutes

Total Time: Approximately 1 hour 20 minutes

Yield:

Serves 4-6

Nutritional Value:

Average nutritional values per serving:

- Calories: 180 kcal

- Protein: 3g

- Carbohydrates: 20g

- Fat: 11g

- Fiber: 6g

Alternative Ingredients:

- For added taste, sprinkle some crumbled feta cheese on top before serving.

Try different veggies, such as carrots or mushrooms, in your experiments.

3. Spanish Patatas Bravas (Spicy Potatoes)

Ingredients:

- 4 large potatoes, peeled and cubed

- 4 tablespoons olive oil

- 2 cloves garlic, minced

- 1 teaspoon smoked paprika

- 1/2 teaspoon cayenne pepper (adjust to taste)

- 1/2 cup tomato sauce or canned diced tomatoes

- 2 tablespoons mayonnaise

- Salt to taste

- Chopped fresh parsley for garnish

Procedure:

1. Aim for 425°F (220°C) in the oven.

2. Cubed potatoes should be evenly coated after being tossed in two tablespoons of olive oil in a basin.

3. Arrange the potatoes evenly on a parchment paper-lined baking pan. Bake for 30 to 35 minutes, or until golden brown and crispy.

4. Heat the final two tablespoons of olive oil in a different pan. Garlic, minced, and sauté until aromatic.

5. Add the diced tomatoes or tomato sauce, cayenne pepper, smoked paprika, and salt. For a few minutes, simmer.

6. Place the baked potatoes in a platter for serving. Over them, drizzle the hot sauce and dollop of mayonnaise.

7. Add freshly chopped parsley as a garnish and serve patatas bravas right away.

Time Frame:

Preparation Time: 15 minutes

Cooking Time: 30-35 minutes

Total Time: Approximately 45-50 minutes

Yield:

Serves 4-6

Nutritional Value:

Average nutritional values per serving:

- Calories: 220 kcal

- Protein: 3g

- Carbohydrates: 30g

- Fat: 10g

- Fiber: 4g

Alternative Ingredients:

- For a variation in flavor, drizzle over some hot sauce with a tomato basis or aioli.

provide a dash of ground cumin to provide another taste dimension.

4. Lebanese Stuffed Zucchini (Kousa Mahshi)

Ingredients:

- 6-8 zucchinis

- 1 cup rice, rinsed

- 1 lb ground beef or lamb

- 1 onion, finely chopped

- 2 tomatoes, finely chopped

- 2 tablespoons tomato paste

- 1/4 cup chopped fresh parsley

- 1/4 cup chopped fresh mint

- 1 teaspoon ground cinnamon

- 1 teaspoon allspice

- Salt and pepper to taste

- Olive oil

- 4 cups chicken or vegetable broth

Procedure:

1. Slice off the tops of the zucchinis and remove the inner flesh by hollowing them out. Keep the hollowed-out zucchinis aside.

2. Combine washed rice, ground lamb or beef, chopped tomatoes, chopped onion, chopped parsley, chopped fresh mint, ground cinnamon, ground allspice, salt, and pepper in a bowl.

3. Load the mixture into the hollowed-out zucchinis, allowing some room for the rice to swell on top.

4. The stuffed zucchini should be put in a saucepan. Pour over them some chicken or veggie broth and drizzle with olive oil.

5. After bringing to a boil, lower the heat, cover, and simmer until the rice and zucchini are cooked, 30 to 40 minutes.

6. Heat up Kousa Mahshi.

Time Frame:

Preparation Time: 30 minutes

Cooking Time: 30-40 minutes

Total Time: Approximately 1 hour 10 minutes

Yield:

Serves 6-8

Nutritional Value:

Average nutritional values per serving:

- Calories: 290 kcal

- Protein: 15g

- Carbohydrates: 25g

- Fat: 15g

-Fiber: 4g

Alternative Ingredients:

- To provide more protein and a different texture, try substituting quinoa for rice.

- For variation, add pine nuts or raisins to the stuffing.

5. Turkish Imam Bayildi (Stuffed Eggplant)

Ingredients:

- 4 small eggplants

- 1 onion, finely chopped

- 3 tomatoes, finely chopped

- 3 cloves garlic, minced

- 1/4 cup chopped fresh parsley

- 1/4 cup chopped fresh mint

- 1 teaspoon ground cumin

- 1 teaspoon paprika

- 1/4 cup olive oil

- Salt and pepper to taste

Procedure:

1. Turn the oven on to 375°F, or 190°C.

2. Split the eggplants lengthwise in half, then remove a portion of the flesh, leaving the shell in place. Keep the flesh you scooped out aside.

3. Warm up some olive oil in a pan over medium heat. Cut onion and sauté till tender. When aromatic, add the minced garlic and sauté it.

4. Add the diced tomatoes, paprika, ground cumin, reserved eggplant flesh, salt, and pepper. Cook until the mixture thickens, a few minutes.

5. Add the chopped fresh mint and parsley and stir.

6. Place the prepared mixture inside the eggplant halves.

7. The filled eggplants should be put on a baking dish. Add a little extra olive oil drizzled on.

8. Bake the eggplants for 35 to 40 minutes, covered with foil, or until they are soft.

9. Serve heated Imam Bayildi.

Time Frame:

Preparation Time: 20 minutes

Cooking Time: 35-40 minutes

Total Time: Approximately 55-60 minutes

Yield:

Serves 4

Nutritional Value:

Average nutritional values per serving:

- Calories: 180 kcal

- Protein: 3g

- Carbohydrates: 20g

- Fat: 11g

- Fiber: 8g

Alternative Ingredients:

- For extra texture, add breadcrumbs or pine nuts to the stuffing.

- Before serving, add a dollop of Greek yogurt on top for a creamy touch.

6. Italian Grilled Mediterranean Vegetables

Ingredients:

- 2 zucchinis, sliced lengthwise

- 2 eggplants, sliced

- 2 bell peppers (red and yellow), halved

- 1 red onion, sliced

- 1/4 cup olive oil

- 2 tablespoons balsamic vinegar

- 2 cloves garlic, minced

- 1 teaspoon dried oregano

- Salt and pepper to taste

- Chopped fresh basil for garnish

Procedure:

1. Grill at a medium-high temperature.

2. Sliced zucchini, eggplants, bell peppers cut in half, red onion slices, olive oil, balsamic vinegar, minced garlic, dried oregano, salt, and pepper should all be combined in a bowl and well coated.

3. The vegetables should be grilled for 3–4 minutes on each side to get soft and browned.

4. Take off of the grill and place on a dish for serving.

5. Before serving, garnish with finely chopped fresh basil.

Time Frame:

Preparation Time: 15 minutes

Cooking Time: 8-10 minutes

Total Time: Approximately 25 minutes

Yield:

Serves 4-6

Nutritional Value:

Average nutritional values per serving:

- Calories: 120 kcal

- Protein: 2g

- Carbohydrates: 15g

- Fat: 7g

- Fiber: 5g

Alternative Ingredients:

- For added zest, add a drizzle of lemon juice or a scattering of crumbled feta cheese.

-Try different veggies, such as mushrooms or cherry tomatoes.

7. Greek Spanakopita (Spinach Pie)

Ingredients:

- 1 pound fresh spinach, chopped

- 1 onion, finely chopped

- 3 cloves garlic, minced

- 1/2 cup fresh dill, chopped

- 1/4 cup fresh parsley, chopped

- 1/2 cup feta cheese, crumbled

- 1/2 cup ricotta cheese

- 1/4 cup grated Parmesan cheese

- 1/4 cup olive oil

- 1 package phyllo dough sheets (thawed if frozen)

- Salt and pepper to taste

Procedure:

1. Set oven temperature to 175°C/350°F.

2. Warm up some olive oil in a pan over medium heat. Minced garlic and diced onion should be sautéed till tender.

3. Cook the chopped spinach until it wilts. Turn off the heat and let it cool.

4. Combine the cooked spinach mixture with grated Parmesan cheese, crumbled feta cheese, ricotta cheese, chopped fresh dill, and chopped fresh parsley in a bowl. Season with salt and pepper.

5. Spread some olive oil on a baking dish. Arrange the phyllo sheets in half, smearing a little olive oil on each layer.

6. Cover the layered phyllo sheets with the spinach and cheese mixture.

7. Add the remaining phyllo sheets on top, smearing some olive oil on each layer.

8. With a sharp knife, delicately score the top into squares or triangles.

9. Cook for 40 to 45 minutes, or until well-browned.

10. To serve, let it cool somewhat.

Time Frame:

Preparation Time: 30 minutes

Cooking Time: 40-45 minutes

Total Time: Approximately 1 hour 15 minutes

Yield:

Serves 6-8

Nutritional Value:

Average nutritional values per serving:

- Calories: 250 kcal

- Protein: 8g

- Carbohydrates: 20g

- Fat: 15g

- Fiber: 3g

Alternative Ingredients:

- For a taste change, incorporate a sprinkling of red pepper flakes or a hint of nutmeg.

- If necessary, replace fresh spinach with frozen spinach that has been well-drained.

8. Moroccan Zaalouk (Eggplant and Tomato Dip)

Ingredients:

- 2 large eggplants

- 3 tomatoes, chopped

- 3 cloves garlic, minced

- 1 teaspoon ground cumin

- 1 teaspoon paprika

- 1/4 cup olive oil

- 2 tablespoons chopped fresh parsley

- Salt and pepper to taste

- Lemon wedges for garnish

Procedure:

1. Turn the oven on to 400°F, or 200°C. After scoring the eggplants with a fork, roast them for 45 to 50 minutes on a baking sheet, or until they are soft.

2. After allowing the roasted eggplants to cool, remove the skin and cut the flesh.

3. Warm up some olive oil in a pan over medium heat. Garlic, minced, and sauté until aromatic.

4. Add the chopped paprika, tomatoes, and roasted eggplants, along with the salt, pepper, and cumin. Cook, slightly mashing the mixture, for 15 to 20 minutes.

5. Add the fresh parsley and stir. Cook for a further five minutes.

6. Zaalouk can be served cold or room temperature, topped with

Time Frame:

Preparation Time: 10 minutes

Cooking Time: 70-75 minutes

Total Time: Approximately 1 hour 25 minutes

Yield:

Serves 4-6

Nutritional Value:

Average nutritional values per serving:

- Calories: 120 kcal

- Protein: 2g

- Carbohydrates: 10g

- Fat: 8g

- Fiber: 5g

Alternative Ingredients:

- Incorporate a pinch of cayenne pepper for a hint of spiciness.

- Add a tablespoon of vinegar or lemon juice for a tangy flavor.

9. Spanish Escalivada (Roasted Vegetables)

Ingredients:

- 2 large red bell peppers

- 2 large eggplants

- 2 large onions

- 4 cloves garlic, unpeeled

- 1/4 cup olive oil

- Salt to taste

- Chopped fresh parsley for garnish

Procedure:

1. Aim for 425°F (220°C) in the oven. Arrange on a baking sheet the whole red bell peppers, eggplants, onions, and peeled garlic cloves.

2. After the vegetables are soft and the skins are browned, roast them for 45 to 50 minutes.

3. Take them out of the oven and allow them to cool a little.

4. Remove the peel off the eggplants and bell peppers. Cut the veggies into thin strips.

5. Place the cut veggies in an arrangement on a serving dish. Salt and olive oil should be drizzled on.

6. Before serving, sprinkle some freshly chopped parsley on top.

Time Frame:

Preparation Time: 10 minutes

Cooking Time: 45-50 minutes

Total Time: Approximately 55-60 minutes

Yield:

Serves 4-6

Nutritional Value:

Average nutritional values per serving:

- Calories: 100 kcal

- Protein: 2g

- Carbohydrates: 10g

- Fat: 7g

- Fiber: 5g

Alternative Ingredients:

- Utilize a blend of red and yellow bell peppers to introduce further hue variance.

- For an added zest, drizzle with balsamic vinegar or a little lemon juice.

10. Lebanese Fattoush Salad

Ingredients:

- 4 pita bread rounds, toasted and torn into pieces

- 2 tomatoes, diced

- 1 cucumber, diced

- 1 red onion, thinly sliced

- 1 green bell pepper, diced

- 1 cup chopped fresh parsley

- 1/2 cup chopped fresh mint

- 1/4 cup olive oil

- 1/4 cup lemon juice

- 2 cloves garlic, minced

- 1 teaspoon sumac (optional)

- Salt and pepper to taste

Procedure:

1. Tears of pita bread, diced tomatoes, diced cucumber, red onion, diced green bell pepper, chopped parsley, and chopped mint should all be combined in a big bowl.

2. To create the dressing, combine olive oil, lemon juice, minced garlic, sumac (if desired), salt, and pepper in a different bowl.

3. Over the salad, drizzle with the dressing and toss lightly to mix.

4. To allow the flavors to mix, let the salad sit for ten to fifteen minutes.

5. Serve the Fattoush Salad right away.

Time Frame:

Preparation Time: 15 minutes

Total Time: Approximately 15-20 minutes

Yield:

Serves 4-6

Nutritional Value:

Average nutritional values per serving:

- Calories: 180 kcal

- Protein: 4g

- Carbohydrates: 20g

- Fat: 10g

- Fiber: 4g

Alternative Ingredients:

- For added crunch, add chopped lettuce or diced radishes.

- Add pomegranate seeds on top for a colorful and sweet pop.

1. Greek Grilled Octopus

Ingredients:

- 1 octopus (about 2-3 pounds), cleaned and tenderized

- 1/2 cup olive oil

- 3 cloves garlic, minced

- Juice of 2 lemons

- 2 tablespoons fresh oregano, chopped

- Salt and pepper to taste

- Lemon wedges for serving

Procedure:

1. Heat up a big saucepan of water until it boils. When the octopus is cooked, add it and simmer for 30 to 40 minutes.

2. After taking it out of the water, allow the octopus to cool. Turn the grill's heat to high.

3. Combine olive oil, lemon juice, chopped fresh oregano, minced garlic, salt, and pepper in a bowl.

4. After putting the octopus on the grill, spray it with the olive oil mixture and cook it for four to five minutes on each side.

5. After taking it from the grill, cut the octopus into portions for serving. Accompany with wedges of lemon.

Time Frame:

Preparation Time: 15 minutes

Cooking Time: 35-45 minutes

Total Time: Approximately 50-60 minutes

Yield:

Serves 4-6

Nutritional Value:

Average nutritional values per serving:

- Calories: 180 kcal

- Protein: 20g

- Carbohydrates: 2g

- Fat: 10g

- Fiber: 0g

Alternative Ingredients:

- For a distinct citrus flavor, use lime juice instead of lemon.

For a little kick of heat, add a scattering of crushed red pepper flakes.

2. Italian Cioppino (Seafood Stew)

Ingredients:

- 2 tablespoons olive oil

- 1 onion, chopped

- 3 cloves garlic, minced

- 1 fennel bulb, sliced

- 1 red bell pepper, diced

- 1 can (28 oz) crushed tomatoes

- 2 cups seafood or fish stock

- 1 cup dry white wine

- 1 teaspoon dried oregano

- 1 teaspoon dried thyme

- Salt and pepper to taste

- 1 pound mixed seafood (such as shrimp, clams, mussels, squid, fish fillets)

- Chopped fresh parsley for garnish

Procedure:

1. Heat the olive oil in a big pot or Dutch oven over medium heat. Minced garlic and diced onion should be sautéed till tender.

2. Add the diced red bell pepper and the sliced fennel. Cook until just beginning to soften, a few minutes.

3. Add the crushed tomatoes, dry white wine, dried thyme, dried oregano, and salt and pepper. You can also add shellfish or fish stock. Simmer for twenty to twenty-five minutes.

4. After adding the mixed seafood to the pot, boil it for a further five to eight minutes, or until the seafood is thoroughly cooked.

5. Before serving, sprinkle some freshly chopped parsley on top.

Time Frame:

Preparation Time: 15 minutes

Cooking Time: 35-40 minutes

Total Time: Approximately 50-55 minutes

Yield:

Serves 4-6

Nutritional Value:

Average nutritional values per serving:

- Calories: 250 kcal

- Protein: 25g

- Carbohydrates: 15g

- Fat: 8g

- Fiber: 3g

Alternative Ingredients:

- Utilize several fish types according on personal choice.

- For improved flavor and color, add a small pinch of saffron threads.

3. Spanish Garlic Shrimp (Gambas al Ajillo)

Ingredients:

- 1 pound large shrimp, peeled and deveined

- 6 cloves garlic, thinly sliced

- 1/4 cup olive oil

- 2 tablespoons butter

- 1 teaspoon red pepper flakes (adjust to taste)

- 2 tablespoons chopped fresh parsley

- Salt to taste

- Crusty bread for serving

Procedure:

1. In a large skillet, melt butter and olive oil over medium heat. Add the red pepper flakes and the thinly sliced garlic. Sauté the garlic until it becomes yellow, but not burnt.

2. Put the shrimp in the skillet and turn the heat up to medium-high. Cook until pink, 2 to 3 minutes on each side.

3. Add salt and freshly chopped parsley on top. To mix, toss.

4. Accompany the steaming Gambas al Ajillo with a fresh toast.

Time Frame:

Preparation Time: 10 minutes

Cooking Time: 5-6 minutes

Total Time: Approximately 15-16 minutes

Yield:

Serves 4

Nutritional Value:

Average nutritional values per serving:

- Calories: 220 kcal

- Protein: 25g

- Carbohydrates: 2g

- Fat: 12g

- Fiber: 0g

Alternative Ingredients:

A dash of dry white wine can add even more flavor depth.

Add some lemon wedges as a garnish for some citrus flavor.

4. Moroccan Fish Tagine with Chermoula

Ingredients:

- 1 1/2 pounds firm white fish fillets (such as cod or halibut), cut into chunks

- 2 tablespoons olive oil

- 1 onion, finely chopped

- 2 tomatoes, diced

- 1 preserved lemon, flesh removed, rind thinly sliced

- 1/2 cup chopped fresh cilantro

- 1/4 cup chopped fresh parsley

- 2 cloves garlic, minced

- 1 teaspoon ground cumin

- 1 teaspoon paprika

- 1 teaspoon ground coriander

- 1/2 teaspoon ground turmeric

- Salt and pepper to taste

- Lemon wedges for serving

Procedure:

1. Mix olive oil, diced tomatoes, finely chopped onion, chopped parsley, thinly sliced preserved lemon rind, minced garlic, ground cumin, paprika, ground coriander, ground turmeric, salt, and pepper in a bowl.

2. Arrange the fish chunks in a deep skillet or tagine. Cover the fish with the prepared mixture.

3. The fish should be cooked thoroughly after 20 to 25 minutes of cooking under cover on low heat.

4. With lemon wedges, serve the Moroccan Fish Tagine hot.

Time Frame:

Preparation Time: 15 minutes

Cooking Time: 20-25 minutes

Total Time: Approximately 35-40 minutes

Yield:

Serves 4

Nutritional Value:

Average nutritional values per serving:

- Calories: 200 kcal

- Protein: 25g

- Carbohydrates: 5g

- Fat: 8g

- Fiber: 2g

Alternative Ingredients:

- For a different herbal touch, use fresh mint leaves in place of fresh cilantro.

- Use freshly grated lemon zest in place of preserved lemon.

5. Greek Baked Lemon-Herb Fish

Ingredients:

- 4 fish fillets (such as snapper or sea bass)

- 1/4 cup olive oil

- Juice of 1 lemon

- 2 cloves garlic, minced

- 2 tablespoons chopped fresh parsley

- 1 tablespoon chopped fresh dill

- Salt and pepper to taste

- Lemon slices for garnish

Procedure:

1. Turn the oven on to 375°F, or 190°C. Fish fillets should be put on a baking dish.

2. Mix olive oil, lemon juice, minced garlic, chopped fresh dill, chopped fresh parsley, salt, and pepper in a basin.

3. Evenly coat the fish fillets by pouring the mixture over them.

4. Fish should flake easily with a fork and be cooked through after baking for 15 to 20 minutes.

5. Before serving, garnish with slices of lemon.

Time Frame:

Preparation Time: 10 minutes

Cooking Time: 15-20 minutes

Total Time: Approximately 25-30 minutes

Yield:

Serves 4

Nutritional Value:

Average nutritional values per serving:

- Calories: 220 kcal

- Protein: 30g

- Carbohydrates: 1g

- Fat: 10g

- Fiber: 0g

Alternative Ingredients:

- Replace dill with thyme or basil for a different herb flavor.

- Drizzle with a touch of honey for a hint of sweetness.

6. Italian Linguine with Clams

Ingredients:

- 1 pound linguine pasta

- 3 pounds fresh clams, scrubbed

- 1/4 cup olive oil

- 4 cloves garlic, minced

- 1/2 teaspoon red pepper flakes (adjust to taste)

- 1/2 cup dry white wine

- 1/4 cup chopped fresh parsley

- Salt to taste

Procedure:

1. Follow the directions on the package to cook the linguine pasta in a big pot of boiling salted water. After draining, set away.

2. Heat the olive oil in a big skillet over medium heat. Add the red pepper flakes and minced garlic. Add the garlic and sauté until golden, but not browned.

3. After the clams have been cleaned, add dry white wine to the skillet. Once the clams open, heat them covered for five to seven minutes.

4. Throw away any unopened clams. Add the chopped fresh parsley and cooked linguine noodles. Add salt to taste to season. Gently toss to mix.

5. Warm linguine with clams is served.

Time Frame:

Preparation Time: 15 minutes

Cooking Time: 15-20 minutes

Total Time: Approximately 30-35 minutes

Yield:

Serves 4-6

Nutritional Value:

Average nutritional values per serving:

- Calories: 400 kcal

- Protein: 20g

- Carbohydrates: 60g

- Fat: 10g

- Fiber: 3g

Alternative Ingredients:

- Garnish with grated Parmesan cheese or a squeeze of lemon juice for added flavor.

7. Spanish Grilled Sardines (Sardinas a la Parrilla)

Ingredients:

- 8 fresh sardines, cleaned and gutted

- 1/4 cup olive oil

- 2 cloves garlic, minced

- 2 tablespoons chopped fresh parsley

- 1 tablespoon lemon juice

- Salt and pepper to taste

Procedure:

1. Grill at a medium-high temperature.

2. Combine olive oil, lemon juice, chopped fresh parsley, minced garlic, salt, and pepper in a bowl.

3. Evenly coat the sardines by brushing them with the olive oil mixture.

4. The sardines should be cooked through and have a slight sear after grilling for three to four minutes on each side.

5. Take off of the grill and serve warm.

Time Frame:

Preparation Time: 10 minutes

Cooking Time: 6-8 minutes

Total Time: Approximately 15-18 minutes

Yield:

Serves 4

Nutritional Value:

Average nutritional values per serving:

- Calories: 180 kcal

- Protein: 20g

- Carbohydrates: 0g

- Fat: 10g

- Fiber: 0g

Alternative Ingredients:

- Add a sprinkle of smoked paprika for an extra layer of flavor.

- Serve with a side of grilled vegetables or a fresh salad.

Ingredients:

- 4 salmon fillets

- 2 tablespoons olive oil

- 1 tablespoon ground cumin

- 1 tablespoon paprika

- 1 teaspoon ground coriander

- 1 teaspoon ground cinnamon

- 1/2 teaspoon ground ginger

- Salt and pepper to taste

- Lemon wedges for serving

Procedure:

1. Turn the oven on to 400°F, or 200°C. Arrange the salmon fillets on a parchment paper-lined baking pan.

2. Combine olive oil, salt, pepper, ground ginger, ground cinnamon, ground paprika, ground coriander, and ground cumin in a bowl.

3. Evenly coat the salmon fillets by brushing them with the spice mixture.

4. Bake the salmon for 12 to 15 minutes, or until it's cooked through and flake readily when tested with a fork.

5. Serve warm Moroccan Spiced Salmon with wedges of lemon.

Time Frame:

Preparation Time: 10 minutes

Cooking Time: 12-15 minutes

Total Time: Approximately 25 minutes

Yield:

Serves 4

Nutritional Value:

Average nutritional values per serving:

- Calories: 250 kcal

- Protein: 30g

- Carbohydrates: 1g

- Fat: 12g

- Fiber: 0g

Alternative Ingredients:

- Substitute ground cinnamon with a pinch of ground cloves for a different spice blend.

- Drizzle with honey or maple syrup for a touch of sweetness.

9. Greek Shrimp Saganaki

Ingredients:

- 1 pound large shrimp, peeled and deveined

- 2 tablespoons olive oil

- 1 onion, finely chopped

- 3 cloves garlic, minced

- 1 can (14 oz) diced tomatoes

- 1/2 cup crumbled feta cheese

- 1/4 cup chopped fresh parsley

- 1 teaspoon dried oregano

- 1 tablespoon ouzo or brandy (optional)

- Salt and pepper to taste

Procedure:

1. In a skillet over medium heat, warm the olive oil. Minced garlic and finely chopped onion should be sautéed till tender.

2. To the skillet, add diced tomatoes together with their liquid. Cook for five to seven minutes.

3. Add large shrimp, salt, pepper, dried oregano, chopped fresh parsley, crumbled feta cheese, and ouzo or brandy (if using). Cook until the shrimp are well cooked, about 8 to 10 minutes.

4. Garnish the hot shrimp saganaki with more chopped parsley.

Time Frame:

Preparation Time: 15 minutes

Cooking Time: 15-20 minutes

Total Time: Approximately 30-35 minutes

Yield:

Serves 4

Nutritional Value:

Average nutritional values per serving:

- Calories: 220 kcal

- Protein: 25g

- Carbohydrates: 6g

- Fat: 10g

- Fiber: 1g

Alternative Ingredients:

- Substitute ouzo or brandy with a splash of white wine for a different flavor profile.

- Add a pinch of chili flakes for a hint of spiciness.

10. Italian Tuscan-Style Grilled Swordfish

Ingredients:

- 4 swordfish steaks

- 1/4 cup balsamic vinegar

- 2 tablespoons olive oil

- 4 cloves garlic, minced

- 2 tablespoons chopped fresh rosemary

- Salt and pepper to taste

- Lemon wedges for serving

Procedure:

1. Combine olive oil, balsamic vinegar, chopped fresh rosemary, minced garlic, salt, and pepper in a bowl.

2. Evenly cover the swordfish steaks by brushing them with the marinade. Give them 20 to 30 minutes to marinade.

3. Grill at a medium-high temperature. Sear the swordfish steaks for 5 to 6 minutes on each side, or until done.

4. Warm Tuscan-Style Grilled Swordfish is served with wedges of lemon.

Time Frame:

Preparation Time: 10 minutes

Marinating Time: 20-30 minutes

Cooking Time: 10-12 minutes

Total Time: Approximately 40-52 minutes

Yield:

Serves 4

Nutritional Value:

Average nutritional values per serving:

- Calories: 300 kcal

- Protein: 35g

- Carbohydrates: 2g

- Fat: 15g

- Fiber: 0g

Alternative Ingredients:

- Replace rosemary with thyme or basil for a different herbaceous flavor.

- Drizzle with a balsamic reduction for added richness.

1. Spanish Chicken and Chorizo Paella

Ingredients:

- 4 bone-in chicken thighs

- 6 oz chorizo sausage, sliced

- 1 onion, chopped

- 2 cloves garlic, minced

- 1 red bell pepper, diced

- 1 tomato, diced

- 1 1/2 cups Arborio rice

- 3 1/2 cups chicken broth

- 1 teaspoon smoked paprika

- 1 teaspoon saffron threads (optional)

- 1 cup frozen peas

- Salt and pepper to taste

- Lemon wedges for serving

Procedure:

1. Brown the chorizo slices and chicken thighs in a big skillet or paella pan. Take out and place aside.

2. Diced tomato, diced red bell pepper, minced garlic, and chopped onion should all be sautéed until soft.

3. Add the saffron threads (if using), Arborio rice, and smoked paprika and stir. Simmer for one minute.

4. After adding the chicken broth, boil the mixture. Return the chorizo and browned chicken thighs to the pan.

5. Cook, stirring periodically, for 15 to 20 minutes. During the final five minutes of cooking, add the frozen peas.

6. Add pepper and salt for seasoning. With lemon wedges, serve hot Paella with chicken and chorizo.

Time Frame:

Preparation Time: 15 minutes

Cooking Time: 30-35 minutes

Total Time: Approximately 45-50 minutes

Yield:

Serves 4-6

Nutritional Value:

Average nutritional values per serving:

- Calories: 450 kcal

- Protein: 25g

- Carbohydrates: 40g

- Fat: 20g

- Fiber: 3g

Alternative Ingredients:

- Use smoked paprika for a deeper flavor.

- Add shrimp or mussels for a seafood twist.

2. Greek Lemon-Herb Roast Chicken

Ingredients:

- 1 whole chicken (about 4-5 pounds)

- 1/4 cup olive oil

- Juice of 2 lemons

- Zest of 1 lemon

- 3 cloves garlic, minced

- 2 teaspoons dried oregano

- 1 teaspoon dried thyme

- Salt and pepper to taste

- Fresh rosemary sprigs for garnish

Procedure:

1. Turn the oven on to 375°F, or 190°C. After rinsing, blot the chicken dry with paper towels.

2. Olive oil, lemon juice, zest, minced garlic, dried oregano, dried thyme, salt, and pepper should all be combined in a bowl.

3. Apply the prepared mixture all over the chicken.

4. Transfer the chicken to a baking dish or roasting pan. Bake for one and a half to one and a half hours, or until the internal temperature reaches 165°F (74°C).

5. Give the chicken ten minutes to rest before slicing. Garnish with sprigs of fresh rosemary.

Time Frame:

Preparation Time: 10 minutes

Cooking Time: 1 hour 15 minutes to 1 hour 30 minutes

Total Time: Approximately 1 hour 25 minutes to 1 hour 40 minutes

Yield:

Serves 4-6

Nutritional Value:

Average nutritional values per serving:

- Calories: 300 kcal

- Protein: 35g

- Carbohydrates: 2g

- Fat: 16g

- Fiber: 0g

Alternative Ingredients:

- Replace dried herbs with fresh herbs for a stronger aroma.

- Add slices of lemon under the chicken skin for extra citrus flavor.

3. Italian Osso Buco (Braised Veal Shanks)

Ingredients:

- 4 veal shanks

- 1/2 cup all-purpose flour

- 4 tablespoons olive oil

- 1 onion, chopped

- 2 carrots, chopped

- 2 stalks celery, chopped

- 4 cloves garlic, minced

- 1 can (14 oz) diced tomatoes

- 1 cup beef or veal stock

- 1/2 cup dry white wine

- 2 sprigs fresh thyme

- 2 bay leaves

- Gremolata (chopped parsley, garlic, and lemon zest) for garnish

Procedure:

1. After adding salt and pepper to the veal shanks, coat them with flour and shake off any excess.

2. In a big pot or Dutch oven, warm up the olive oil over medium-high heat. Shanks of brown veal on all sides. Take out and place aside.

3. Add the minced garlic, diced onion, chopped carrots, and chopped celery to the same saucepan and sauté until softened.

4. Add Bay leaves, fresh thyme sprigs, dry white wine, diced tomatoes, and beef or veal stock. Put the veal shanks back in the pot.

5. After bringing it to a boil, turn down the heat. The veal should be tender after 2–1/2 hours of simmering under cover.

6. Serve the hot Osso Buco with gremolata on top.

Time Frame:

Preparation Time: 20 minutes

Cooking Time: 2-2 1/2 hours

Total Time: Approximately 2 hours 20 minutes to 2 hours 50 minutes

Yield:

Serves 4

Nutritional Value:

Average nutritional values per serving:

- Calories: 400 kcal

- Protein: 30g

- Carbohydrates: 10g

- Fat: 20g

- Fiber: 2g

Alternative Ingredients:

- Substitute veal shanks with beef shanks for a different taste.

- Add a splash of balsamic vinegar for depth of flavor.

4. Moroccan Chicken Couscous with Raisins and Almonds

Ingredients:

- 4 chicken thighs

- 1 onion, finely chopped

- 2 cloves garlic, minced

- 1 teaspoon ground cumin

- 1 teaspoon ground coriander

- 1/2 teaspoon ground cinnamon

- 1/2 teaspoon ground turmeric

- 1 cup chicken broth

- 1 cup couscous

- 1/4 cup raisins

- 1/4 cup slivered almonds

- Fresh cilantro for garnish

- Salt and pepper to taste

Procedure:

1. Add salt, pepper, ground cumin, ground coriander, ground cinnamon, and ground turmeric to the chicken thighs for seasoning.

2. Chicken thighs should be browned in a big skillet. Take out and place aside.

3. Finely chopped onion and minced garlic should be sautéed until transparent.

4. Simmer the chicken stock after adding it to the skillet. Place the chicken thighs back in the skillet.

5. Add the raisins, slivered almonds, and couscous and stir. To ensure the couscous is soft, cook it covered for 8 to 10 minutes.

6. Present Moroccan Chicken.Hot couscous with a fresh cilantro garnish.

Time Frame:

Preparation Time: 15 minutes

Cooking Time: 20-25 minutes

Total Time: Approximately 35-40 minutes

Yield:

Serves 4

Nutritional Value:

Average nutritional values per serving:

- Calories: 350 kcal

- Protein: 25g

- Carbohydrates: 30g

- Fat: 15g

- Fiber: 4g

Alternative Ingredients:

- Add chopped dried apricots for a sweeter flavor.

- Substitute almonds with pine nuts for a nutty twist.

5. Lebanese Kafta Kebabs

Ingredients:

- 1 pound ground lamb or beef

- 1 onion, finely chopped

- 2 cloves garlic, minced

- 1/4 cup chopped fresh parsley

- 1 teaspoon ground cumin

- 1 teaspoon ground coriander

- 1/2 teaspoon ground cinnamon

- Salt and pepper to taste

- Skewers for grilling

Procedure:

1. Combine minced garlic, finely chopped onion, chopped fresh parsley, ground cumin, ground coriander, ground cinnamon, salt, and pepper in a bowl with ground lamb or beef.

2. Wrap the mixture around skewers to form lengthy, sausage-like kebabs.

3. For 8 to 10 minutes, over medium-high heat, grill the Kafta Kebabs, turning them regularly, until they are cooked through and browned.

4. Serve warm pita bread, salad, or rice alongside Lebanese kafta kebabs.

Time Frame:

Preparation Time: 15 minutes

Cooking Time: 8-10 minutes

Total Time: Approximately 25 minutes

Yield:

Serves 4

Nutritional Value:

Average nutritional values per serving:

- Calories: 280 kcal

- Protein: 25g

- Carbohydrates: 3g

- Fat: 18g

- Fiber: 1g

Alternative Ingredients:

- Incorporate chopped mint leaves for a refreshing taste.

- Add a pinch of sumac for an extra layer of flavor.

6. Turkish Chicken Kebabs (Tavuk Şiş)

Ingredients:

- 1 1/2 pounds boneless, skinless chicken breasts, cut into cubes

- 1/4 cup olive oil

- 3 tablespoons plain yogurt

- 2 cloves garlic, minced

- 1 teaspoon paprika

- 1 teaspoon ground cumin

- 1 teaspoon ground coriander

- Juice of 1 lemon

- Salt and pepper to taste

- Skewers for grilling

Procedure:

1. Olive oil, plain yogurt, paprika, minced garlic, ground cumin, ground coriander, lemon juice, salt, and pepper should all be combined in a bowl.

2. Coat the cubed chicken equally with the marinade. Let the food marinate for a minimum of two hours, or better yet, overnight.

3. Grill at a medium-high temperature. Put chicken that has been marinated on skewers.

4. The chicken kebabs should be cooked through and gently browned after 10 to 12 minutes of grilling, with periodic turning.

5. Serve warm Turkish Chicken Kebabs with flatbread, salad, or rice.

Time Frame:

Preparation Time: 15 minutes (+ marinating time)

Cooking Time: 10-12 minutes

Total Time: Approximately 25-27 minutes (+ marinating time)

Yield:

Serves 4

Nutritional Value:

Average nutritional values per serving:

- Calories: 280 kcal

- Protein: 35g

- Carbohydrates: 2g

- Fat: 14g

- Fiber: 1g

Alternative Ingredients:

- Substitute chicken breasts with boneless thighs for a different texture.

- Add a pinch of red pepper flakes for a hint of spiciness.

7. Italian Tuscan-Style Grilled Pork Chops

Ingredients:

- 4 bone-in pork chops

- 1/4 cup olive oil

- 2 cloves garlic, minced

- 2 tablespoons chopped fresh rosemary

- Zest of 1 lemon

- Salt and pepper to taste

Procedure:

1. Combine olive oil, lemon zest, minced garlic, chopped fresh rosemary, salt, and pepper in a bowl.

2. Coat the pork chops uniformly by rubbing them with the mixture. Give them half an hour to marinate.

3. Grill at a medium-high temperature. Cook the pork chops on the grill for 4–5 minutes on each side, or until done.

4. Before serving, let the Tuscan-Style Grilled Pork Chops a few minutes to rest.

Time Frame:

Preparation Time: 10 minutes (+ marinating time)

Cooking Time: 8-10 minutes

Total Time: Approximately 18-20 minutes (+ marinating time)

Yield:

Serves 4

Nutritional Value:

Average nutritional values per serving:

- Calories: 320 kcal

- Protein: 35g

- Carbohydrates: 0g

- Fat: 20g

- Fiber: 0g

Alternative Ingredients:

- Replace fresh rosemary with dried rosemary, using half the quantity.

- Serve with a squeeze of lemon juice for added freshness.

8. Greek Lamb Souvlaki with Tzatziki

Ingredients for Lamb Souvlaki:

- 1 1/2 pounds lamb leg or shoulder, cut into cubes

- 1/4 cup olive oil

- 3 cloves garlic, minced

- 2 tablespoons red wine vinegar

- 1 tablespoon dried oregano

- Juice of 1 lemon

- Salt and pepper to taste

- Skewers for grilling

Ingredients for Tzatziki:

- 1 cup Greek yogurt

- 1 cucumber, grated and squeezed to remove excess moisture

- 2 cloves garlic, minced

- 1 tablespoon olive oil

- 1 tablespoon chopped fresh dill

- Juice of 1/2 lemon

- Salt and pepper to taste

Procedure for Lamb Souvlaki:

1. Olive oil, minced garlic, red wine vinegar, dried oregano, lemon juice, salt, and pepper should all be combined in a bowl.

2. Coat the cubed lamb thoroughly in the marinade. Let it marinate for at least two hours or overnight in the fridge.

3. Lamb that has marinated is skewered. Grill at a medium-high temperature.

4. The lamb souvlaki should be cooked to your preferred doneness after 8 to 10 minutes on the grill, turning them over now and again.

Procedure for Tzatziki:

1. Greek yogurt, grated cucumber, minced garlic, lemon juice, olive oil, chopped fresh dill, and salt and pepper should all be combined in a bowl.

2. Once fully combined, chill until ready to serve.

Time Frame:

Preparation Time (Lamb Souvlaki): 15 minutes (+ marinating time)

Preparation Time (Tzatziki): 10 minutes

Cooking Time (Lamb Souvlaki): 8-10 minutes

Total Time: Approximately 33-35 minutes (+ marinating time)

Yield:

Serves 4

Nutritional Value (Lamb Souvlaki):

Average nutritional values per serving:

- Calories: 340 kcal

- Protein: 30g

- Carbohydrates: 3g

- Fat: 20g

- Fiber: 1g

Nutritional Value (Tzatziki - per serving):

Average nutritional values per serving:

- Calories: 60 kcal

- Protein: 3g

- Carbohydrates: 4g

- Fat: 4g

- Fiber: 0g

Alternative Ingredients:

- Substitute lamb with beef or chicken for different variations.

- For Tzatziki, use mint instead of dill for a unique flavor.

9. Spanish Beef Empanadas

Ingredients for Empanada Dough:

- 3 cups all-purpose flour

- 1 teaspoon salt

- 1/2 cup cold unsalted butter, diced

- 1 egg

- 1/2 cup cold water

Ingredients for Filling:

- 1 pound ground beef

- 1 onion, finely chopped

- 2 cloves garlic, minced

- 1 teaspoon ground cumin

- 1 teaspoon paprika

- 1/2 teaspoon chili powder (optional)

- 1/4 cup chopped green olives

- Salt and pepper to taste

- Olive oil for cooking

Procedure for Empanada Dough:

1. Combine salt and all-purpose flour in a big bowl. Blend in the chopped cold butter until it resembles coarse crumbs.

2. Add the egg and cold water to the flour mixture after beating them together. Work the dough until it comes together. Gently knead until it forms a ball. After covering, chill for half an hour.

Procedure for Filling:

1. Heat the olive oil in a pan over medium heat. Minced garlic and finely chopped onion should be sautéed till tender.

2. Cook the ground beef until it turns brown. Add chopped green olives, paprika, ground cumin, chili powder (if using), salt, and pepper. Simmer for an additional five minutes. Turn off the heat and let it to cool.

Assembling Empanadas:

1. Turn the oven on to 375°F, or 190°C. Use parchment paper to line baking sheets.

2. Spread the cooled dough onto a surface dusted with flour. Cut out circles with a diameter of roughly 5 to 6 inches.

3. Spoon some of the beef filling that has cooled down into the center of each dough round. Shape the dough into a half-moon by folding it over the filling. Using a fork to press, seal the edges.

4. Line the baking sheets with the prepared empanadas. Use a beaten egg to brush the tops.

5. Bake for 20 to 25 minutes, or until golden brown, in a preheated oven.

Time Frame:

Preparation Time (Dough): 10 minutes (+ chilling time)

Preparation Time (Filling): 15 minutes

Assembly Time: 20 minutes

Baking Time: 20-25 minutes

Total Time: Approximately 65-70 minutes (+ chilling time)

Yield:

Makes 12 empanadas

Nutritional Value (per empanada):

Average nutritional values per serving:

- Calories: 250 kcal

- Protein: 12g

- Carbohydrates: 20g

- Fat: 13g

- Fiber: 1g

Alternative Ingredients:

- Use ground chicken or turkey instead of beef.

- Add raisins or chopped bell peppers to the filling for extra flavors.

Absolutely! Here's a more concise version of the Moroccan Lamb Tagine with Apricots and Almonds:

Ingredients:

- 2 pounds lamb shoulder, cut into chunks

- 2 onions, finely chopped

- 3 cloves garlic, minced

- 1 teaspoon ground ginger

- 1 teaspoon ground cumin

- 1 teaspoon ground coriander

- 1/2 teaspoon ground cinnamon

- 1/2 teaspoon saffron threads (optional)

- 1 cup dried apricots, halved

- 1/2 cup blanched almonds

- 2 cups chicken or vegetable broth

- 2 tablespoons olive oil

- Salt and pepper to taste

- Fresh cilantro for garnish

Procedure:

1. In a large saucepan or tagine with a heavy bottom, heat the olive oil over medium heat. Lamb chunks should be brown in batches until browned. Put aside.

2. Saute the chopped onions in the same pot until they become tender. Add the minced garlic and heat for an additional one minute.

3. Put the browned lamb back in the pot. Add the ground ginger, coriander, cumin, cinnamon, and, if using, saffron threads, along with the salt and pepper. To thoroughly mix in the spices, coat the meat and onions.

4. Cover the meat with the vegetable or chicken broth. Once it reaches a boil, lower the heat to a simmer. Cook the lamb covered for one and a half to two hours, or until it is tender.

5. To the tagine, add the blanched almonds and dried apricots. Simmer for a further 20 to 30 minutes, or until the flavors combine and the apricots swell up.

6. Modify the seasoning as needed. Before serving, garnish with fresh cilantro.

7. Warm couscous or toast should be served with the Moroccan Lamb Tagine with Apricots & Almonds.

Time Frame:

Preparation Time: 20 minutes

Cooking Time: 2-2.5 hours

Total Time: Approximately 2.5-3 hours

Yield:

Serves 4-6

Nutritional Value:

Average nutritional values per serving:

- Calories: 450 kcal

- Protein: 30g

- Carbohydrates: 25g

- Fat: 25g

- Fiber: 5g

Alternative Ingredients:

- Use prunes or raisins instead of apricots for a different sweetness.

- Replace almonds with pine nuts for a distinct nutty flavor.

1. Spanish Tortilla Española

Ingredients:

- 4-5 medium potatoes, peeled and thinly sliced

- 1 onion, thinly sliced

- 6 eggs

- Salt and pepper to taste

- Olive oil for frying

Procedure:

1. In a big skillet over medium heat, warm up the olive oil. Add the onions and potatoes, cut thinly. Potatoes should be cooked slowly until they are soft but not browned. With the oil reserved, drain the potatoes and onions.

2. Beat the eggs and add salt and pepper to taste in a bowl. Gently stir in the onions and the drained potatoes.

3. Warm up a small amount of the set-aside oil in a non-stick skillet. Add the egg mixture to the potato mixture.

4. Cook until the bottom sets, about 5 to 7 minutes on low heat. After covering the skillet with a plate, turn the tortilla back into it. Cook until well done, 5 to 7 more minutes.

5. Transfer the Tortilla Española onto a plate for serving. Cut into wedges and serve warm or at room temperature.

Time Frame:

Preparation Time: 15-20 minutes

Cooking Time: 15-20 minutes

Total Time: Approximately 30-40 minutes

Yield:

Serves 4-6

Nutritional Value:

Average nutritional values per serving:

- Calories: 220 kcal

- Protein: 10g

- Carbohydrates: 20g

- Fat: 10g

- Fiber: 3g

Alternative Ingredients:

- Add diced bell peppers or chorizo for extra flavor.

- Replace regular potatoes with sweet potatoes for a twist.

2. Greek Spanakopita (Spinach and Feta Pie)

Ingredients:

- 1 pound fresh spinach, chopped

- 1 bunch fresh dill, finely chopped

- 1 bunch fresh parsley, finely chopped

- 1 onion, finely chopped

- 8 ounces feta cheese, crumbled

- 4 eggs, beaten

- 1/2 cup olive oil

- 10 phyllo pastry sheets

- Salt and pepper to taste

Procedure:

1. Set oven temperature to 175°C/350°F. Coat a baking dish in oil.

2. Add chopped spinach and onion to a pan and cook until wilted. Pour off extra liquid and allow to cool.

3. Combine the feta cheese crumbles, chopped dill, parsley, beaten eggs, cooled spinach mixture, olive oil, salt, and pepper in a bowl.

4. Brush each sheet of phyllo pastry with olive oil before layering half of them in the baking dish that has been buttered. Evenly distribute the spinach and cheese mixture.

5. Brush each sheet of phyllo with olive oil before arranging the remaining sheets on top.

6. Using a sharp knife, gently score the top into squares or triangles.

7. Bake for 45 to 50 minutes, or until golden brown, in a preheated oven.

8. Before dividing the Spanakopita into parts, let it cool somewhat.

Time Frame:

Preparation Time: 30 minutes

Cooking Time: 45-50 minutes

Total Time: Approximately 75-80 minutes

Yield:

Serves 6-8

Nutritional Value:

Average nutritional values per serving:

- Calories: 280 kcal

- Protein: 10g

- Carbohydrates: 20g

- Fat: 18g

- Fiber: 3g

Alternative Ingredients:

- Substitute fresh spinach with frozen, thawed, and drained spinach.

- Incorporate mint leaves for an additional layer of flavor.

3. Italian Frittata with Mixed Vegetables

Ingredients:

- 6 eggs

- 1 cup mixed vegetables (bell peppers, zucchini, tomatoes, etc.), diced

- 1 onion, finely chopped

- 1/4 cup grated Parmesan cheese

- 2 tablespoons olive oil

- Salt and pepper to taste

Procedure:

1. Set oven temperature to 175°C/350°F.

2. Heat the olive oil in an ovenproof skillet over medium heat. Add the chopped onion and sauté until the vegetables are soft. Add pepper and salt for seasoning.

3. Beat eggs in a bowl and add grated Parmesan cheese. Over the skillet of sautéed vegetables, pour the egg mixture.

4. Cook for 3–4 minutes on medium heat, or until the edges are set. After preheating the oven, move the skillet inside.

5. The frittata should be set and golden brown after 10 to 12 minutes in the oven.

6. Take it out of the oven and let it a few minutes to cool down before slicing.

7. The Italian Frittata can be served warm or room temperature.

Time Frame:

Preparation Time: 10-15 minutes

Cooking Time: 15-20 minutes

Total Time: Approximately 25-35 minutes

Yield:

Serves 4-6

Nutritional Value:

Average nutritional values per serving:

- Calories: 150 kcal

- Protein: 10g

- Carbohydrates: 5g

- Fat: 10g

- Fiber: 2g

Alternative Ingredients:

- Add cooked bacon or ham for a meatier variation.

- Incorporate fresh herbs like basil or thyme for extra aroma.

4. Moroccan Shakshuka

Ingredients:

- 1 tablespoon olive oil

- 1 onion, finely chopped

- 2 cloves garlic, minced

- 1 bell pepper, diced

- 1 teaspoon ground cumin

- 1 teaspoon paprika

- 1/2 teaspoon ground cayenne pepper (adjust to taste)

- 1 can (14 oz) diced tomatoes

- 4-6 eggs

- Salt and pepper to taste

- Fresh cilantro or parsley for garnish

Procedure:

1. In a skillet over medium heat, warm the olive oil. Sauté the chopped onion until it turns transparent.

2. Add the diced bell pepper and minced garlic. Cook until peppers become tender.

3. Add the ground cayenne pepper, paprika, and cumin. Stir until aromatic, about one minute.

4. Add the chopped tomatoes together with their juices. Simmer the sauce for ten to fifteen minutes, or until it slightly thickens.

5. Crack the eggs into the little wells you've made in the sauce. To cook the eggs to the desired doneness (runny or set), cover the skillet.

6. Add salt and pepper to the Shakshuka to season it. Add some fresh parsley or cilantro as a garnish.

7. Serve hot straight out of the skillet with pita or crusty bread.

Time Frame:

Preparation Time: 10 minutes

Cooking Time: 20-25 minutes

Total Time: Approximately 30-35 minutes

Yield:

Serves 2-4

Nutritional Value:

Average nutritional values per serving:

- Calories: 200 kcal

- Protein: 10g

- Carbohydrates: 12g

- Fat: 12g

- Fiber: 4g

Alternative Ingredients:

- Include diced chorizo or feta cheese for added flavor variations.

- Adjust the spice level by increasing or decreasing cayenne pepper.

5. Lebanese Eggplant Fatteh

Ingredients:

- 2 medium eggplants, sliced

- 2 cups plain yogurt

- 2 cloves garlic, minced

- 1 cup cooked chickpeas

- 1 cup pita chips or toasted pita bread, broken into pieces

- 1/4 cup pine nuts, toasted

- 2 tablespoons olive oil

- 1 teaspoon ground cumin

- Salt and pepper to taste

- Chopped fresh parsley for garnish

Procedure:

1. Turn the oven on to 400°F, or 200°C. Arrange the slices of eggplant on a baking sheet, coat them with olive oil, and sprinkle with salt and pepper. Roast until soft, 20 to 25 minutes.

2. Combine plain yogurt, minced garlic, and a dash of salt in a bowl. Put aside.

3. Heat the olive oil in a pan over medium heat. Add the ground cumin and cooked chickpeas. Cook for a few minutes, or until thoroughly heated.

4. Place the slices of roasted eggplant in a serving plate. Add toasted pita slices and cooked chickpeas on top.

5. Evenly distribute the garlic yogurt mixture throughout the layers.

6. Top with chopped fresh parsley and toasted pine nuts.

7. Warm Lebanese eggplant fatah should be served.

Time Frame:

Preparation Time: 15-20 minutes

Cooking Time: 20-25 minutes

Total Time: Approximately 35-45 minutes

Yield:

Serves 4-6

Nutritional Value:

Average nutritional values per serving:

- Calories: 280 kcal

- Protein: 8g

- Carbohydrates: 30g

- Fat: 15g

- Fiber: 7g

Alternative Ingredients:

- Use roasted cauliflower or zucchini as a substitute for eggplant.

- Drizzle with tahini sauce for extra flavor.

6. Turkish Menemen (Scrambled Eggs with Tomatoes)

Ingredients:

- 4 eggs

- 4 tomatoes, chopped

- 1 onion, finely chopped

- 1 green pepper, finely chopped

- 2 tablespoons olive oil

- 1 teaspoon red pepper flakes (optional)

- Salt and pepper to taste

- Fresh parsley for garnish

Procedure:

1. In a skillet over medium heat, warm the olive oil. Add the green pepper and onion, chopped. Sauté the food until it becomes tender.

2. When the tomatoes are chopped and start to release their juices, add them to the skillet and simmer.

3. Add salt, pepper, and red pepper flakes (if using). Blend thoroughly.

4. Straight into the tomato mixture, crack eggs. Gently whisk the eggs until they are little runny but still scrambled.

5. Take it off the heat source and give it a minute or two to rest.

6. Before serving, garnish with fresh parsley.

Time Frame:

Preparation Time: 10 minutes

Cooking Time: 10-15 minutes

Total Time: Approximately 20-25 minutes

Yield:

Serves 2-3

Nutritional Value:

Average nutritional values per serving:

- Calories: 180 kcal

- Protein: 10g

- Carbohydrates: 10g

- Fat: 12g

- Fiber: 3g

Alternative Ingredients:

- Add chopped sausage or Turkish sucuk for a heartier dish.

- Include chopped spinach or feta cheese for a twist.

7. Italian Eggs in Purgatory (Uova in Purgatorio)

Ingredients:

- 4 eggs

- 2 cups tomato sauce

- 2 cloves garlic, minced

- 1 teaspoon red pepper flakes (adjust to taste)

- 2 tablespoons olive oil

- Fresh basil leaves for garnish

- Grated Parmesan cheese (optional)

- Salt and pepper to taste

Procedure:

1. In a skillet over medium heat, warm the olive oil. Add the red pepper flakes and minced garlic. For one minute, sauté.

2. Transfer the sauce verde to the skillet. Simmer until slightly thickened, 5 to 7 minutes.

3. Crack eggs into wells you've made in the sauce. Add salt and pepper to the eggs for seasoning.

4. For about five to seven minutes, or until the eggs are set but the yolks are still runny, cover the skillet and cook the eggs.

5. If preferred, garnish with grated Parmesan cheese and fresh basil leaves.

6. Serve the Purgatory Eggs right out of the skillet.

Time Frame:

Preparation Time: 5 minutes

Cooking Time: 15-20 minutes

Total Time: Approximately 20-25 minutes

Yield:

Serves 2-4

Nutritional Value:

Average nutritional values per serving:

- Calories: 180 kcal

- Protein: 10g

- Carbohydrates: 10g

- Fat: 12g

- Fiber: 2g

Alternative Ingredients:

- Add diced bell peppers or Italian sausage for variation.

- Use marinara sauce instead of tomato sauce for different flavors.

8. Greek Eggplant Moussaka

Ingredients:

- 2 large eggplants, sliced

- 1 pound ground lamb or beef

- 1 onion, finely chopped

- 2 garlic cloves, minced

- 2 cups tomato sauce

- 1 teaspoon ground cinnamon

- 1 teaspoon dried oregano

- 1/2 cup grated Parmesan cheese

- 1/4 cup breadcrumbs

- 2 tablespoons olive oil

- Salt and pepper to taste

- Bechamel Sauce:

  - 3 tablespoons butter

  - 1/4 cup all-purpose flour

  - 2 cups milk

  - 1/2 cup grated Parmesan cheese

  - Pinch of nutmeg

  - Salt and pepper to taste

- Fresh parsley for garnish

Procedure:

1. Turn the oven on to 375°F, or 190°C. Slices of eggplant should be brushed with olive oil and baked for 20 to 25 minutes, or until soft. Put aside.

2. Heat the olive oil in a pan over medium heat. Add minced garlic and diced onion. Sauté the food until it becomes tender.

3. Cook the ground lamb (or beef) in the skillet until it turns brown. Eliminate extra fat.

4. Add tomato sauce, salt, pepper, ground cinnamon, and dry oregano. Simmer for a duration of 15 to 20 minutes.

5. To make the Bechamel Sauce, melt the butter in a pot over a medium heat. Whisk in flour until smooth. Milk should be added gradually while whisking continuously to thicken the sauce. Take off the heat and mix in the nutmeg, salt, pepper, and grated Parmesan cheese.

6. Arrange half of the eggplant slices in a baking dish. Cover the eggplant with the meat mixture. Arrange the remaining eggplant pieces in another layer.

7. Over the layered eggplant and meat mixture, pour the Bechamel Sauce. Top with grated Parmesan cheese and breadcrumbs.

8. Bake for 35 to 40 minutes, or until golden brown, in a preheated oven.

9. Before serving the Greek Eggplant Moussaka, sprinkle some fresh parsley on top.

Time Frame:

Preparation Time: 30 minutes

Cooking Time: 1 hour 20 minutes

Total Time: Approximately 1 hour 50 minutes

Yield:

Serves 6-8

Nutritional Value:

Average nutritional values per serving:

- Calories: 380 kcal

- Protein: 20g

- Carbohydrates: 20g

- Fat: 25g

- Fiber: 6g

Alternative Ingredients:

- Substitute ground meat with lentils for a vegetarian version.

- Use zucchini slices alongside or instead of eggplant for a variation.

9. Spanish Huevos Rotos (Broken Eggs with Potatoes)

Ingredients:

- 4 large potatoes, peeled and thinly sliced

- 4 eggs

- 4 cloves garlic, minced

- 1/4 cup olive oil

- Salt and pepper to taste

- Chopped fresh parsley for garnish

Procedure:

1. In a skillet over medium heat, warm the olive oil. Saute the minced garlic until it turns yellow, without burning it. Take out and place the garlic aside.

2. Fry the thinly sliced potatoes in the same skillet until they are crispy and golden brown. Use paper towels to absorb surplus oil. Add pepper and salt for seasoning.

3. Fry the eggs (over-easy or sunny-side up) in a separate pan.

4. Place the fried potatoes onto a platter for dishing. Top with the fried eggs.

5. Over the eggs and potatoes, scatter the saved sautéed garlic.

6. Drizzle the Spanish Huevos Rotos with finely chopped fresh parsley before serving.

Time Frame:

Preparation Time: 15-20 minutes

Cooking Time: 20-25 minutes

Total Time: Approximately 35-45 minutes

Yield:

Serves 4

Nutritional Value:

Average nutritional values per serving:

- Calories: 320 kcal

- Protein: 10g

- Carbohydrates: 25g

- Fat: 20g

- Fiber: 4g

Alternative Ingredients:

- Add sliced chorizo or ham for a meaty variation.

- Top with melted cheese for extra richness.

10. Moroccan Berber Omelet with Herbs

Ingredients:

- 6 eggs

- 1 onion, finely chopped

- 2 tomatoes, diced

- 1/4 cup chopped fresh parsley

- 1/4 cup chopped fresh cilantro

- 2 tablespoons olive oil

- Salt and pepper to taste

Procedure:

1. In a skillet over medium heat, warm the olive oil. Chop the onion and sauté it until transparent.

2. Cook the diced tomatoes until they become tender.

3. Beat the eggs in a basin. Add the chopped fresh cilantro and parsley, as well as the salt and pepper. Blend thoroughly.

4. Transfer the egg mixture into the skillet that contains the tomatoes and onions.

5. Swirl the pan occasionally while cooking the omelet to ensure the eggs solidify but remain slightly runny in the center.

6. After dividing the omelet in half, place it on a serving plate.

7. Warm Moroccan Berber Omelet should be served.

Time Frame:

Preparation Time: 10-15 minutes

Cooking Time: 10-15 minutes

Total Time: Approximately 20-30 minutes

Yield:

Serves 2-3

Nutritional Value:

Average nutritional values per serving:

- Calories: 180 kcal

- Protein: 10g

- Carbohydrates: 5g

- Fat: 12g

- Fiber: 2g

Alternative Ingredients:

- Incorporate diced bell peppers or spinach for added texture and flavor.

- Sprinkle feta cheese on top for a different taste.

1. Italian Margherita Pizza

Ingredients:

- Pizza dough (store-bought or homemade)

- 1 cup tomato sauce

- 8 oz fresh mozzarella cheese, sliced

- Fresh basil leaves

- Olive oil

- Salt and pepper to taste

Procedure:

1. Set oven temperature to 475°F (245°C). When the oven is preheating, put the pizza stone in.

2. On a surface dusted with flour, roll out the pizza dough to the appropriate thickness.

3. Evenly distribute the tomato sauce on the dough.

4. Place fresh mozzarella slices over the sauce.

5. To taste, add salt and pepper for seasoning.

6. Over the pizza, drizzle a little olive oil.

7. Bake for 12 to 15 minutes, or until the cheese is bubbling and beginning to brown and the crust is golden.

8. When ready to serve, remove from the oven and sprinkle fresh basil leaves on top.

Time Frame:

Preparation Time: 10-15 minutes (plus time for dough preparation if homemade)

Cooking Time: 12-15 minutes

Total Time: Approximately 25-30 minutes

Yield:

Makes 1 large pizza

Alternative Ingredients:

- Add thinly sliced tomatoes or cherry tomatoes for extra freshness.

- Incorporate a sprinkle of grated Parmesan cheese or a drizzle of balsamic glaze for added flavor.

2. Turkish Lahmacun (Turkish Pizza)

Ingredients:

For the Dough:

- 3 cups all-purpose flour

- 1 cup warm water

- 2 tablespoons olive oil

- 1 teaspoon salt

- 1 teaspoon sugar

- 1 packet dry yeast

For the Topping:

- 1/2 pound ground lamb or beef

- 1 onion, finely chopped

- 2 tomatoes, finely chopped

- 2 tablespoons tomato paste

- 2 tablespoons olive oil

- 2 teaspoons paprika

- 1 teaspoon ground cumin

- 1 teaspoon ground cinnamon

- Salt and pepper to taste

- Fresh parsley for garnish

- Lemon wedges

Procedure:

1. Mix the flour, sugar, salt, olive oil, warm water, and dry yeast to make the dough. Mix it until a nice dough is formed. For one hour, cover and allow it to rise.

2. Set oven temperature to 475°F (245°C).

3. Roll out the dough thinly after dividing it into smaller balls.

4. Combine the ground beef, chopped tomatoes, chopped onion, chopped olive oil, paprika, ground cumin, ground cinnamon, salt, and pepper in a bowl to make the topping.

5. Over the rolled-out dough, evenly distribute the topping mixture.

6. Bake for 10 to 12 minutes in a preheated oven, or until the meat is cooked through and the sides are golden brown.

7. Add some fresh parsley as a garnish and serve with wedges of lemon for squeezing.

Time Frame:

Preparation Time: 20-30 minutes (plus dough rising time)

Cooking Time: 10-12 minutes

Total Time: Approximately 30-45 minutes

Yield:

Makes 4-6 Lahmacun

Alternative Ingredients:

- Experiment with different meats such as ground chicken or turkey.

- Add chopped bell peppers or chili flakes for a spicier version.

3. Greek Pita Bread with Tzatziki

Ingredients:

For the Pita Bread:

- 2 1/2 cups all-purpose flour

- 1 cup warm water

- 2 tablespoons olive oil

- 1 teaspoon salt

- 1 teaspoon sugar

- 1 packet dry yeast

For the Tzatziki:

- 1 cup Greek yogurt

- 1 cucumber, grated and drained

- 2 cloves garlic, minced

- 1 tablespoon olive oil

- 1 tablespoon lemon juice

- 1 tablespoon chopped fresh dill

- Salt and pepper to taste

Procedure:

Pita Bread:

1. Mix together flour, sugar, salt, warm water, olive oil, and dried yeast. Mix it until a nice dough is formed. For one hour, cover and allow it to rise.

2. Turn the oven on to 500°F, or 260°C.

3. Roll out the smaller dough balls into circles after dividing them into them.

4. Bake for 5 to 7 minutes on a baking sheet, or until they are lightly brown and puffed.

5. Take them out of the oven and, to keep them soft, cover with a cloth.

Tzatziki:

1. In a bowl, combine Greek yogurt, finely chopped fresh dill, grated and drained cucumber, minced garlic, olive oil, and lemon juice. Season with salt and pepper.

2. Let it cool for a minimum of half an hour before serving.

Time Frame:

Preparation Time: 20-30 minutes (plus dough rising time)

Cooking Time: 5-7 minutes

Total Time: Approximately 30-40 minutes

Yield:

Makes 6-8 Pita Breads

Alternative Ingredients:

- Use mint instead of dill in the tzatziki for a different flavor profile.

- Add a pinch of paprika or cumin to the tzatziki for extra depth.

4. Moroccan Khobz (Traditional Bread)

Ingredients:

- 4 cups bread flour

- 1 tablespoon active dry yeast

- 1 tablespoon sugar

- 1 teaspoon salt

- Warm water (as needed)

- Olive oil (for brushing)

Procedure:

1. Mix the bread flour, sugar, salt, and active dry yeast together in a large mixing bowl. Add the warm water little by little and knead the dough until it becomes smooth.

2. Once the dough has doubled in size, cover it and let it rise in a warm location for approximately one hour.

3. Turn the oven on to 450°F, or 230°C.

4. The risen dough should be pounded down and divided into smaller balls. Create a spherical form by flattening each ball.

5. Transfer the rounds to a parchment paper-lined baking sheet. Lightly apply olive oil to the tops.

6. Bake for 15 to 20 minutes, or until the bread is hollow to the touch and is golden brown.

7. The Moroccan Khobz should cool on a wire rack before serving.

Time Frame:

Preparation Time: 15-20 minutes (plus dough rising time)

Cooking Time: 15-20 minutes

Total Time: Approximately 30-40 minutes

Yield:

Makes 4-6 loaves

Alternative Ingredients:

- Sprinkle sesame seeds or nigella seeds on top before baking for added texture and flavor.

- Add a teaspoon of ground cumin or coriander to the dough for a fragrant variation.

5. Italian Focaccia with Rosemary and Sea Salt

Ingredients:

- 4 cups bread flour

- 2 teaspoons active dry yeast

- 1 1/2 cups warm water

- 1/4 cup olive oil (plus extra for drizzling)

- 1 tablespoon sugar

- 2 teaspoons salt

- Fresh rosemary leaves

- Coarse sea salt

Procedure:

1. Combine sugar, active dry yeast, and bread flour in a sizable mixing bowl as well as salt. Add the olive oil and warm water gradually. Mix it until a nice dough is formed.

2. Once the dough has doubled in size, cover it and let it rest in a warm location for one to two hours.

3. Aim for 425°F (220°C) in the oven. A baking sheet can be lined with parchment paper or greased.

4. Place the risen dough onto the baking sheet that has been ready. Form the dough into a square or rectangle by pressing it.

5. Make dimples in the dough by poking it all around with your fingertips. Add a drizzle of olive oil, coarse sea salt, and fresh rosemary leaves.

6. Bake for 20 to 25 minutes, or until the outside is crispy and golden brown.

7. Before slicing and serving the Italian Focaccia, allow it to cool somewhat.

Time Frame:

Preparation Time: 15-20 minutes (plus dough rising time)

Cooking Time: 20-25 minutes

Total Time: Approximately 35-45 minutes

Yield:

Makes 1 large Focaccia

Alternative Ingredients:

- Top the focaccia with cherry tomatoes, olives, or thinly sliced onions for extra flavor and color.

- Sprinkle grated Parmesan or Pecorino cheese on top before baking for a cheesy variation.

6. Lebanese Manakish (Flatbread with Za'atar)

Ingredients:

For the Dough:

- 3 cups all-purpose flour

- 1 cup warm water

- 2 tablespoons olive oil

- 1 teaspoon salt

- 1 teaspoon sugar

- 1 packet dry yeast

For the Topping:

- 1/4 cup za'atar spice mix

- 1/4 cup olive oil

Procedure:

1. Mix the flour, sugar, salt, olive oil, warm water, and dry yeast to make the dough. Mix it until a nice dough is formed. For one hour, cover and allow it to rise.

2. Set oven temperature to 475°F (245°C).

3. Roll out the smaller dough balls into flat circles after dividing them into them.

4. Combine the olive oil and za'atar spice mix. Apply this blend onto the dough that has been rolled out.

5. For 10 to 12 minutes, or until the dough is cooked through and the sides are brown, bake the manakish in a preheated oven.

6. Warm Lebanese Manakish should be served.

Time Frame:

Preparation Time: 20-30 minutes (plus dough rising time)

Cooking Time: 10-12 minutes

Total Time: Approximately 30-45 minutes

Yield:

Makes 4-6 Manakish

Alternative Ingredients:

- Use a combination of herbs like thyme, oregano, and sesame seeds if za'atar spice mix is unavailable.

- Drizzle with a little pomegranate molasses for a tangy kick.

7. Spanish Pan con Tomate (Tomato Bread)

Ingredients:

- 1 loaf of crusty bread (baguette or similar)

- 2-3 ripe tomatoes, halved

- 2 garlic cloves, peeled

- Extra virgin olive oil

- Salt

Procedure:

1. Toast crusty bread slices until they start to turn golden.

2. Apply the sliced side of the garlic cloves to the toasted bread.

3. After removing the skins, rub the halves tomatoes over the bread to distribute the pulp.

4. Pour extra virgin olive oil on top of the bread dipped in tomatoes.

5. Give each slice a small pinch of salt.

6. Serve the Pan with Tomate Spanish style right away.

Time Frame:

Preparation Time: 5-10 minutes

Cooking Time: 5 minutes (toasting)

Total Time: Approximately 10-15 minutes

Yield:

Makes several slices, depending on the size of the bread loaf

Alternative Ingredients:

- Add a sprinkle of Spanish paprika for a hint of smokiness.

- Top with finely chopped fresh herbs like parsley or basil for added freshness.

8. Turkish Pide Bread with Cheese and Herbs

Ingredients:

For the Dough:

- 3 cups all-purpose flour

- 1 cup warm water

- 2 tablespoons olive oil

- 1 teaspoon salt

- 1 teaspoon sugar

- 1 packet dry yeast

For the Topping:

- 1 cup crumbled feta cheese

- 1/4 cup chopped fresh parsley

- 1/4 cup chopped fresh mint

- 2 tablespoons olive oil

Procedure:

1. Mix the flour, sugar, salt, olive oil, warm water, and dry yeast to make the dough. Mix it until a nice dough is formed. For one hour, cover and allow it to rise.

2. Set oven temperature to 475°F (245°C).

3. Roll out the smaller dough balls into oval shapes after dividing them into them.

4. Combine olive oil, chopped fresh mint, chopped fresh parsley, and crumbled feta cheese. Apply this blend onto the dough that has been rolled out.

5. Pide should be baked for 12 to 15 minutes in a preheated oven, or until the dough is cooked through and the edges are brown.

6. Warm Turkish Pide Bread should be served.

Time Frame:

Preparation Time: 20-30 minutes (plus dough rising time)

Cooking Time: 12-15 minutes

Total Time: Approximately 30-45 minutes

Yield:

Makes 4-6 Pide Breads

Alternative Ingredients:

- Substitute feta with another crumbly cheese like goat cheese or ricotta.

- Incorporate sun-dried tomatoes or black olives for additional flavors.

9. Greek Olive Bread

Ingredients:

- 3 cups all-purpose flour

- 1 cup warm water

- 2 tablespoons olive oil

- 1 teaspoon salt

- 1 teaspoon sugar

- 1 packet dry yeast

- 1 cup chopped mixed olives (Kalamata, green, etc.)

- 2 tablespoons chopped fresh rosemary

Procedure:

1. Mix the flour, sugar, salt, olive oil, warm water, and dry yeast to make the dough. Mix it until a nice dough is formed. For one hour, cover and allow it to rise.

2. Set oven temperature to 475°F (245°C).

3. Knead in the fresh rosemary and chopped olives after punching down the raised dough.

4. Roll the dough into a circular loaf and transfer it to a parchment paper-lined baking pan.

5. Use a sharp knife to cut a slit in the top of the bread.

6. Bake for 25 to 30 minutes in a preheated oven, or until the bread is golden brown and hollow to the touch.

7. Before slicing, let the Greek Olive Bread to cool on a wire rack.

Time Frame:

Preparation Time: 20-30 minutes (plus dough rising time)

Cooking Time: 25-30 minutes

Total Time: Approximately 45-60 minutes

Yield:

Makes 1 loaf

Alternative Ingredients:

- Add chopped nuts (like walnuts or almonds) for added texture and taste.

- Use dried herbs like oregano or thyme if fresh rosemary is unavailable.

10. Italian Calzone with Spinach and Ricotta

Ingredients:

For the Dough:

- 3 cups all-purpose flour

- 1 cup warm water

- 2 tablespoons olive oil

- 1 teaspoon salt

- 1 teaspoon sugar

- 1 packet dry yeast

For the Filling:

- 2 cups chopped fresh spinach

- 1 cup ricotta cheese

- 1 cup shredded mozzarella cheese

- 1/4 cup grated Parmesan cheese

- 2 cloves garlic, minced

- Salt and pepper to taste

- 1 egg (for egg wash)

Procedure:

1. Mix the flour, sugar, salt, olive oil, warm water, and dry yeast to make the dough. Mix it until a nice dough is formed. Shut it off and allow it to rise for One hour.

2. Set oven temperature to 475°F (245°C).

3. Combine chopped fresh spinach, grated Parmesan cheese, ricotta cheese, shredded mozzarella cheese, minced garlic, and salt & pepper in a bowl.

4. Roll out the portions of the rising dough into circles after dividing it into halves.

5. Leaving space on the edges, place the filling on one half of each dough circle. To form a semicircular shape, fold the other half over and crimp the edges to seal.

6. For a golden crust, beat an egg and brush it over the calzones.

7. The calzones should be baked for 12 to 15 minutes in a preheated oven, or until golden brown.

8. Before serving the Italian Calzone with Spinach and Ricotta, let them cool somewhat.

Time Frame:

Preparation Time: 30-40 minutes (plus dough rising time)

Cooking Time: 12-15 minutes

Total Time: Approximately 45-60 minutes

Yield:

Makes 4-6 Calzones

Alternative Ingredients:

- Add chopped sun-dried tomatoes or caramelized onions to the filling for extra flavor.

- Incorporate cooked Italian sausage or diced ham for a meatier variation.

1. Greek Honey and Yogurt Parfait with Fresh Fruits

Ingredients:

- 2 cups Greek yogurt

- 1/4 cup honey

- Assorted fresh fruits (strawberries, blueberries, bananas, etc.)

- Granola or chopped nuts (optional)

Procedure:

1. Blend honey and Greek yogurt in a bowl until thoroughly blended.

2. Arrange the honey yogurt mixture among fresh fruits in dishes or serving glasses.

3. You might choose to add chopped nuts or granola in between the layers.

4. After layering again, top with a layer of fresh fruit.

5. The Greek Honey and Yogurt Parfait should be served right away.

Time Frame:

Preparation Time: 10-15 minutes

Total Time: Approximately 10-15 minutes

Yield:

Makes 2-4 servings, depending on glass size

Alternative Ingredients:

- Use flavored yogurt like vanilla or strawberry for added variety.

- Top with a drizzle of additional honey or a sprinkle of cinnamon for extra flavor.

2. Italian Tiramisu

Ingredients:

- 1 cup heavy cream

- 1 cup mascarpone cheese

- 3 tablespoons sugar

- 1 teaspoon vanilla extract

- 1 cup strong brewed coffee, cooled

- 2 tablespoons coffee liqueur (optional)

- Ladyfingers (savoiardi)

- Cocoa powder for dusting

Procedure:

1. Beat heavy cream in a mixing bowl until firm peaks form.

2. Beat the mascarpone cheese, sugar, and vanilla extract together until smooth in a separate bowl.

3. Once the mascarpone mixture and whipped cream are thoroughly blended, fold them gently together.

4. In a shallow plate, mix the cooled brewed coffee and coffee liqueur, if using.

5. Make sure the ladyfingers are moistened but not drenched by quickly dipping them into the coffee mixture.

6. Line a serving dish with a layer of soaking ladyfingers.

7. Over the ladyfingers, spread half of the mascarpone mixture.

8. Repeat the layers using the mascarpone mixture and soaked ladyfingers.

9. The Tiramisu should be covered and chilled for at least two to four hours, preferably overnight.

10. Dust the top with a good amount of chocolate powder before serving.

Time Frame:

Preparation Time: 30-40 minutes (plus chilling time)

Total Time: Approximately 2-4 hours (including chilling time)

Yield:

Makes 6-8 servings

Alternative Ingredients:

- Substitute the coffee liqueur with a non-alcoholic coffee syrup or omit it entirely.

- Garnish with chocolate shavings or grated chocolate for added richness.

3. Turkish Baklava

Ingredients:

- 1 package phyllo pastry sheets (about 1 pound)

- 2 cups chopped nuts (pistachios, walnuts, or a mix)

- 1 cup unsalted butter, melted

- 1 cup sugar

- 1 cup water

- 1/2 cup honey

- 1 teaspoon lemon juice

- Ground cinnamon (optional)

Procedure:

1. Set oven temperature to 175°C/350°F.

2. Place a sheet of phyllo pastry in a baking dish that has been greased, then cover it with melted butter.

3. Repeat this process with half of the phyllo sheets and butter layered on top, followed by half of the chopped nuts.

4. Continue to layer the butter and remaining phyllo sheets.

5. Before baking, cut the baklava into square or diamond shapes with a sharp knife.

6. Bake for 45 to 50 minutes in a preheated oven, or until crispy and golden brown.

7. Make the syrup by mixing sugar, water, honey, and lemon juice in a pot while the baklava bakes. Simmer until slightly thickened, 10 to 15 minutes.

8. Pour the hot syrup over the warm baklava as soon as it's finished baking.

9. Before serving, let the baklava cool fully.

Time Frame:

Preparation Time: 30-40 minutes

Cooking Time: 45-50 minutes

Total Time: Approximately 1.5-2 hours

Yield:

Varies based on cut size; approximately 24 pieces

Alternative Ingredients:

- Add a pinch of ground cinnamon to the nut mixture for extra flavor.

- Substitute honey with a simple syrup made with equal parts sugar and water.

4. Spanish Churros with Chocolate Sauce

Ingredients:

- 1 cup water

- 2 tablespoons sugar

- 1/2 teaspoon salt

- 2 tablespoons vegetable oil

- 1 cup all-purpose flour

- Vegetable oil for frying

- 1/4 cup sugar mixed with 1 teaspoon ground cinnamon (for coating)

- Chocolate sauce for dipping

Procedure:

1. Put the vegetable oil, sugar, salt, and water in a saucepan. Heat till boiling.

2. After turning off the heat, stir in the flour. Until the mixture forms a ball, stir it vigorously.

3. In a deep pan, heat the vegetable oil for frying.

4. Transfer the dough into a piping bag that has a star tip attached.

5. Using scissors to cut the dough strips, pipe the strips straight into the heated oil. Fry till the color turns golden brown.

6. Turn the churros out of the oil and pat dry with paper towels.

7. Dredge the warm churros in the mixture of sugar and cinnamon.

8. Present the Spanish Churros beside a chocolate sauce to dip them in.

Time Frame:

Preparation Time: 15-20 minutes

Cooking Time: 15-20 minutes

Total Time: Approximately 30-40 minutes

Yield:

Makes about 15-20 churros

Alternative Ingredients:

- Dip the churros in melted chocolate or caramel sauce for a different flavor.

- Add a pinch of cayenne pepper to the cinnamon-sugar mixture for a spicy kick.

5. Lebanese Muhallabia (Milk Pudding)

Ingredients:

- 4 cups milk

- 1/2 cup sugar

- 1/2 cup cornstarch

- 1 teaspoon rose water (optional)

- Chopped pistachios or almonds for garnish

Procedure:

1. Pour 3.5 cups of milk and sugar into a pot and heat over medium heat, stirring occasionally.

2. Combine cornstarch and the remaining 1/2 cup milk in a small bowl, whisking until smooth.

3. When the milk is heated through but not boiling, gradually add the cornstarch mixture to the pot while stirring all the time.

4. Stirring continually, cook the mixture until it thickens and coats the spoon's back.

5. Take off the heat and, if desired, mix in some rose water.

6. Transfer the pudding into bowls or serving tureens.

7. After letting the Muhallabia cool, chill it for at least one or two hours to solidify.

8. Before serving, garnish with chopped almonds or pistachios.

Time Frame:

Preparation Time: 5-10 minutes

Cooking Time: 10-15 minutes

Chilling Time: 1-2 hours

Total Time: Approximately 1.5-2.5 hours (including chilling time)

Yield:

Makes 4-6 servings

Alternative Ingredients:

- Flavor the pudding with orange blossom water instead of rose water for a different aroma.

- Top with a sprinkle of ground cinnamon or cardamom for additional flavor.

6. Moroccan Orange and Almond Cake (M'hanncha)

Ingredients:

- 2 cups almond flour

- 1 cup granulated sugar

- Zest of 2 oranges

- 4 eggs

- 1 teaspoon baking powder

- 1/2 teaspoon almond extract

- Powdered sugar for dusting

- Sliced almonds for garnish

Procedure:

1. Set oven temperature to 175°C/350°F. Line and grease a cake pan.

2. Almond flour, eggs, baking powder, orange zest, and almond extract should all be combined in a bowl. Blend until thoroughly blended.

3. Transfer the mixture into the ready-made cake pan.

4. A toothpick inserted into the center should come out clean after the cake has baked for 30 to 35 minutes, or until it is golden.

5. Allow the cake to cool fully inside the pan.

6. When the Moroccan Orange and Almond Cake has cooled, sprinkle it with powdered sugar and top it with almond slices for presentation.

Time Frame:

Preparation Time: 10-15 minutes

Baking Time: 30-35 minutes

Total Time: Approximately 40-50 minutes

Yield:

Makes 8-10 servings

Alternative Ingredients:

- Use lemon zest instead of orange zest for a different citrus flavor.

- Drizzle the cooled cake with a simple syrup made from orange juice and sugar for added moisture and flavor.

7. Italian Cannoli with Ricotta and Pistachios

Ingredients:

For the Cannoli Shells:

- 2 cups all-purpose flour

- 2 tablespoons sugar

- 1 tablespoon cocoa powder

- 2 tablespoons butter, softened

- 1 egg yolk

- 1/2 cup sweet Marsala wine

- Vegetable oil for frying

For the Filling:

- 2 cups ricotta cheese

- 1/2 cup powdered sugar

- 1 teaspoon vanilla extract

- 1/2 cup chopped pistachios

Procedure:

1. Mix the flour, sugar, butter, egg yolk, cocoa powder, and Marsala wine together in a bowl. Work the dough until it becomes smooth. Give it a half-hour to relax.

2. Cut the dough into circles by rolling it thinly. Encircle the cannoli tubes or metal shapes with the circles, then use egg wash to seal the edges.

3. The cannoli shells should be fried in hot, vegetable oil until they are golden brown. Once drained, place on paper towels to chill.

4. Combine ricotta cheese, powdered sugar, vanilla essence, and chopped pistachios in a separate bowl and stir until thoroughly blended.

5. The ricotta mixture should be piped into the chilled cannoli shells using a piping bag.

6. Before serving, sprinkle little powdered sugar over the Italian cannoli.

Time Frame:

Preparation Time: 30-40 minutes (plus dough resting time)

Cooking Time: 15-20 minutes

Total Time: Approximately 1-1.5 hours

Yield:

Makes about 12 cannoli

Alternative Ingredients:

- Substitute chopped almonds or chocolate chips for pistachios in the filling.

- Dip the ends of the cannoli in melted chocolate and sprinkle with additional chopped nuts for decoration.

8. Greek Loukoumades (Honey Puffs)

Ingredients:

- 2 cups all-purpose flour

- 1 teaspoon instant yeast

- 1/2 teaspoon salt

- 1 tablespoon sugar

- 1 1/2 cups warm water

- Vegetable oil for frying

- Honey

- Chopped nuts (optional) for garnish

Procedure:

1. Combine flour, sugar, salt, and instant yeast in a bowl. Warm water should be added gradually and mixed until a smooth batter develops. For one hour, cover and allow it to rise.

2. In a big saucepan or pan, heat the vegetable oil.

3. Little quantities of the batter should be dropped into the hot oil with a spoon or scoop and cooked until golden brown.

4. After removing the Loukoumades from the oil, use paper towels to absorb any leftover oil.

5. While still heated, drizzle with honey and, if preferred, top with chopped nuts.

6. Present the Greek Loukoumades right away.

Time Frame:

Preparation Time: 10-15 minutes (plus batter rising time)

Cooking Time: 15-20 minutes

Total Time: Approximately 25-35 minutes

Yield:

Makes about 20-25 Loukoumades

Alternative Ingredients:

- Add a pinch of cinnamon or nutmeg to the batter for extra flavor.

- Sprinkle with powdered sugar or a mix of cinnamon and sugar instead of honey for serving.

9. Spanish Crema Catalana

Ingredients:

- 4 cups milk

- 6 egg yozks

- 1 cup sugar

- Zest of 1 lemon

- 1 cinnamon stick

- 3 tablespoons cornstarch

- Brown sugar for caramelizing

Procedure:

1. Heat the milk in a skillet with the cinnamon stick and lemon zest until it begins to simmer. After turning off the heat, let it steep for fifteen minutes. Put the strainer back on low heat.

2. Beat the egg yolks, sugar, and cornstarch together until smooth in a bowl.

3. Whisk continually as you slowly pour the warm milk over the egg mixture.

4. Put the mixture back in the saucepan and cook, stirring frequently, over medium-low heat until it thickens enough to coat the spoon's back.

5. After turning off the heat, transfer the Crema Catalana to serving mugs. Give it time to cool.

6. The Crema Catalana should be refrigerated for two to three hours, or until set.

7. Evenly dust each serving dish with brown sugar, then use a kitchen torch or broiler to caramelize the sugar.

Time Frame:

Preparation Time: 15-20 minutes (plus chilling time)

Cooking Time: 15-20 minutes

Total Time: Approximately 30-40 minutes (excluding chilling time)

Yield:

Makes 4-6 servings

Alternative Ingredients:

- Replace the lemon zest with orange zest for a variation in citrus flavor.

- Top with fresh berries or a sprinkle of ground cinnamon for serving.

10. Turkish Künefe

Ingredients:

- 1 pound kadayıf dough (shredded phyllo dough)

- 1 cup unsalted cheese (mozzarella or unsalted white cheese like akkawi), shredded

- 1 cup unsalted butter, melted

- Pistachios or chopped nuts for garnish (optional)

Syrup:

- 2 cups sugar

- 1 cup water

- 1 tablespoon lemon juice

- Rose or orange blossom water (optional)

Procedure:

1. First, get the sugar syrup ready. Add the lemon juice, water, and sugar to a saucepan. Bring to a boil and whisk occasionally to dissolve the sugar. Allow the syrup to gently thicken by simmering it for ten to fifteen minutes. Take off the heat and, if you'd like, drizzle in some orange or rose water. Give it time to cool.

2. Set oven temperature to 175°C/350°F. Oil a circular baking dish.

3. Split the dough for kadayıf into two halves. Press half of the dough evenly on the bottom of the prepared pan.

4. Evenly distribute the shredded cheese on top of the dough.

5. Gently press the remaining kadayıf dough onto the surface.

6. Evenly cover the upper layer with melted butter.

7. Bake for 30 to 40 minutes, or until golden brown, in a preheated oven.

8. After baking, take the Künefe out of the oven and quickly cover it with the cooled sugar syrup, letting it soak.

9. Before slicing, let it a few minutes to rest.

10. If desired, garnish with chopped nuts or pistachios.

11. Enjoy and warm up!

Time Frame:

Preparation Time: 30-40 minutes

Cooking Time: 30-40 minutes

Total Time: Approximately 1.5-2 hours

Yield:

Makes 8-10 servings

Alternative Ingredients:

- Substitute the shredded cheese with a mix of mozzarella and mild white cheese for a balanced taste.

- If kadayıf dough is not available, thin angel hair-style vermicelli can be used as a substitute.

Conclusion

Encouraging Healthy Eating Habits in Children:

Promoting wholesome eating practices in kids is essential for their general growth and well-being. The Mediterranean diet provides an excellent foundation for establishing these behaviors at a young age. A foundation for balanced nutrition is established by its emphasis on whole foods, fruits, vegetables, lean proteins, and healthy fats. Introducing kids to a variety of tastes, textures, and nutrient-dense foods can have a big impact on their lifelong dietary preferences and decisions.

Children find the Mediterranean diet appealing because of its versatility, which makes a broad variety of vibrant and savory dishes possible. Getting children involved in meal preparation increases their sense of food ownership and curiosity, which increases their acceptance and enjoyment of healthier options. Including kids in the kitchen fosters a healthy relationship with food and emphasizes the value of a balanced diet, whether through assistance with product selection at the market or basic cooking activities.

Children's nutritional needs are met and new tastes in food are introduced when they are encouraged to eat a variety of fruits, vegetables, complete grains, and lean meats. For instance, you can introduce children to a variety of flavors and textures by having them help prepare Greek salads with feta and olives or by having them eat Italian panzanella (bread salad).

Final Tips and Suggestions for Parents:

1. Lead by Example: Kids are more likely to pick up healthy eating practices if they see their parents doing so. Set an example for your family by introducing Mediterranean-style foods into their regular mealtime routines.

2. Create a Positive Food Environment: Ensure that wholesome meals are easily accessible and abundantly available in your surroundings. To encourage mindful eating and family bonding, encourage family meals together and steer clear of distractions like screens or electronics.

3. Educate Through Experience: Make the most of teaching moments to inform kids about the health advantages of various meals. Describe how particular nutrients are partners in their own nutrition, improving their health and overall well-being.

4. Embrace Moderation: The Mediterranean diet places a strong emphasis on wholesome foods, but it also permits occasional indulgences. Instill in kids the values of moderation and balance, letting them enjoy occasional treats or snacks but making nutrient-dense meals a priority.

5. Encourage Physical Activity: Incorporate an active lifestyle with a nutritious diet. Incorporate enjoyable physical activities for kids into their diet in addition to a balanced diet to promote general wellness, such as sports, outdoor play, or family walks.

Embracing the Mediterranean Lifestyle for Lifelong Wellness:

Living a Mediterranean lifestyle involves more than just diet; it involves many aspects of health. Adopting this lifestyle encourages social and emotional well-being in addition to physical health. The Mediterranean diet places a strong emphasis on long meals, building social bonds, and lowering stress— all of which are beneficial to mental health.

Putting an emphasis on wholesome, fresh foods that are nutrient-dense provides the best possible physical wellness. A lower risk of chronic illnesses like heart disease, obesity, and several types of cancer has been associated with this dietary pattern. By combining aspects of the Mediterranean diet, such as mindful eating, regular exercise, and stress management, one can develop a comprehensive approach to wellness that lasts a lifetime.

Furthermore, the Mediterranean way of life emphasizes the value of social connections and community. Sharing meals with loved ones and friends strengthens social ties and creates a feeling of community, all of which are essential for mental health.

In summary, promoting a Mediterranean diet in kids not only establishes a positive relationship with food but also creates lifelong habits that support general health. Through active participation, exemplary behavior, and highlighting the comprehensive aspects of the Mediterranean diet, parents may enable their kids to make well-informed, health-conscious decisions for a happy and satisfying life.

A. Week 1:

Day 1 - Monday

- **Breakfast:** Greek Yogurt Parfait with Fresh Fruits and Honey

- **Lunch:** Greek Salad with Feta and Olives

- **Dinner:** Spanish Seafood Paella

Day 2 - Tuesday

- **Breakfast:** Whole Grain Toast with Almond Butter and Sliced Banana

- **Lunch:** Italian Pasta e Fagioli

- **Dinner:** Lebanese Kafta Kebabs with Hummus and Tabbouleh

Day 3 - Wednesday

- **Breakfast:** Turkish Menemen (Scrambled Eggs with Tomatoes)

- **Lunch:** Spanish Gazpacho with Whole Grain Bread

- **Dinner:** Greek Lemon-Herb Roast Chicken with Roasted Vegetables

Day 4 - Thursday

- **Breakfast:** Italian Frittata with Mixed Vegetables

- **Lunch:** Moroccan Chickpea and Vegetable Tagine

- **Dinner:** Italian Spaghetti Aglio e Olio with Grilled Mediterranean Vegetables

Day 5 - Friday

- **Breakfast:** Greek Spanakopita (Spinach and Feta Pie)

- **Lunch:** Lebanese Stuffed Zucchini (Kousa Mahshi)

- **Dinner:** Spanish Garlic Shrimp (Gambas al Ajillo) with Patatas Bravas

Day 6 - Saturday

- **Breakfast:** Italian Cannoli with Ricotta and Pistachios

- **Lunch:** Moroccan Harira (Chickpea and Lentil Soup) with Moroccan Orange and Almond Cake for dessert
- **Dinner:** Greek Baked Lemon-Herb Fish with Greek Salad

Day 7 - Sunday
- **Breakfast:** Turkish Pide Bread with Cheese and Herbs
- **Lunch:** Italian Margherita Pizza with a Side Salad
- **Dinner:** Lebanese Chicken Fatteh with Muhallabia for dessert

B. Week 2:

- Incorporate dishes like Tuscan Tomato and Bread Soup (Pappa al Pomodoro), Turkish Bulgur Pilaf with Chickpeas, Greek Pastitsio, Spanish Churros with Chocolate Sauce, and more.

C. Week 3:

- Include meals such as Italian Risotto with Asparagus and Parmesan, Lebanese Freekeh with Chicken and Nuts, Spanish Patatas Bravas, Moroccan Berber Omelet with Herbs, and others.

D. Week 4:

- Integrate recipes such as Greek Pita Bread with Tzatziki, Italian Focaccia with Rosemary and Sea Salt, Moroccan Fish Tagine with Chermoula, Greek Shrimp Saganaki, and more.

The diverse meal plan allows for a rich experience of the Mediterranean diet, exposing children to various flavors, textures, and nutrients across the weeks while ensuring a well-rounded and enjoyable eating experience.